Essential Anaesthesia
for Medical Students

Essential Anaesthesia for Medical Students

Mark PD Heining MD, FRCA

Consultant Anaesthetist, Nottingham City Hospital, and
Honorary Clinical Teacher, Nottingham University Medical School, UK

David G Bogod FRCA

Consultant Anaesthetist, Nottingham City Hospital, and
Honorary Clinical Teacher, Nottingham University Medical School, UK

and

Alan R Aitkenhead MD, FRCA

Professor of Anaesthesia, Nottingham University Medical School,
Queen's Medical Centre, Nottingham, UK

A member of the Hodder Headline Group
LONDON • SYDNEY • AUCKLAND
Co-published in the USA by Oxford University Press, Inc., New York

First published in Great Britain in 1996 by
Arnold, a member of the Hodder Headline Group
338 Euston Road, London NW1 3BH

Co-published in the United States of America by
Oxford University Press, Inc.,
198 Madison Avenue, New York, NY 10016
Oxford is a registered trademark of Oxford University Press

British Library Cataloguing in Publication Data
A catalogue record for this book is available from the British Library

Library of Congress Cataloging-in-Publication Data
A catalog record for this book is available from the Library of Congress

ISBN 0 340 61386 6

Composition by Scribe Design, Gillingham, Kent
Printed and bound in Great Britain by St Edmundsbury Press,
Bury St Edmunds, Suffolk and JW Arrowsmith Ltd, Bristol

Contents

Preface

This book is intended to help undergraduate medical students during their period of attachment to the anaesthetic department. It will complement the teaching which the student receives in theatre, and the lectures and tutorials on anaesthesia which are now part of most medical school courses. To that end, it is designed as a handbook so that it can be consulted at convenient moments on the wards. Mark Heining and David Bogod are Consultant Anaesthetists at the City Hospital, Nottingham and Clinical Teachers at Nottingham University Medical School. Alan Aitkenhead is Professor of Anaesthesia, Nottingham University Medical School, Queen's Medical Centre.

Anaesthesia can appear a mysterious subject, somewhat divorced from the rest of the medical school curriculum. Particularly with the current move towards integrated courses in medical schools, it is important for the student to appreciate that an understanding of anaesthesia is largely a question of applying existing knowledge. The administration of general and regional anaesthesia, as covered in the first two chapters, may be understood readily by applying knowledge of anatomy, physiology and pharmacology. An account of drugs used in anaesthesia is given in the third chapter. Details of practical procedures have been deliberately omitted since these are most effectively dealt with in the operating theatre and anaesthetic room. Anaesthetic apparatus is described so that the student may understand how an anaesthetic is administered safely; monitoring is given a separate chapter because of its important theoretical foundations and because of its increasing applications in other fields of medicine.

Anaesthetists have activities outside the operating theatre, and the second half of the book is devoted to these. The modern medical school curriculum emphasizes the importance of communication and teamwork, and these aspects are emphasized in this section. The pre-operative and post-operative periods may be understood by application of the student's existing knowledge of general medicine and surgery, and liaison with other specialties is emphasized where appropriate. The management of acute post-operative pain is now part of the anaesthetist's workload alongside the established responsibility for the management of patients with chronic intractable pain; these subjects are dealt with in their own chapter, and involve the application of applied pharmacology and anatomy outside the operating theatre. Chapters on intensive care and cardiorespiratory arrest follow, to demonstrate how the same applied sciences, principally pharmacology and physiology, together with a few practical skills, can be used to help the acutely ill patient.

The undergraduate often finds it difficult to apply a knowledge of pre-clinical sciences to clinical subjects. The specialty of anaesthesia offers an ideal opportunity for the student to find this 'missing link' since applied sciences are often easily demonstrable. This book is not intended to teach the undergraduate exactly how to give an anaesthetic; it is not intended to be a house officer's guide to relations with the anaesthetic department; nor is it intended to describe the details of practical procedures. Rather, it is intended to demonstrate to medical undergraduates that apparently complex procedures are largely a question of applying their existing knowledge; to provide a theoretical foundation for their practical discussions in theatre; to emphasize the importance of communication and liaison in clinical decision-making; to help them understand the factors of importance in pre-operative assessment and post-operative management of surgical patients; and, we hope, to make their attachment to the anaesthetic department more enjoyable and fruitful.

PART ONE

The Anaesthetist Inside the Operating Theatre

General Anaesthesia

Introduction

Despite the rise in popularity of local and regional techniques, the term 'anaesthesia' is still regarded by most laymen (and many doctors) as being synonymous with the state of reversible unconsciousness that is produced by general anaesthesia. The debate between the relative merits of general and regional anaesthesia is considered later in this chapter. The anaesthetist is often recognized only as 'the bloke who knocks you out' or 'the gas man'. In fact, the role of the anaesthetist is much more complex, and involves assessment of risk, pre-operative preparation, and keeping the patient alive despite the side-effects of anaesthetic drugs and the excesses of the surgeon during the operation, as well as ensuring that there is no memory of intra-operative events.

History

There has been considerable (and often heated) debate about who deserves the honour of having given the first anaesthetic, and votes are probably evenly split between C.W. Long of Georgia and W.T.G. Morton of Boston, both in the USA. Whatever the truth (and both these gentlemen have reasonable claim), the year was certainly 1846 and ether was the agent used. It is difficult nowadays to appreciate the impact of this simple agent (soon to be rivalled by chloroform in the UK) upon the then barbaric practice of surgery. Due to the appalling trauma suffered during operations, surgery was used as a last resort and the range of procedures limited to those of short duration and obvious benefit, such as amputation of a gangrenous limb. After the introduction of anaesthesia, surgery became a far more acceptable treatment and its practitioners began to rise in status to the pre-eminent position they now hold.

The first anaesthetics were simple enough and chloroform was often used by pouring it onto gauze held near the face, a practice instituted by James Young Simpson in Edinburgh to relieve the pain of childbirth, and later popularized by John Snow, generally regarded as the first professional anaesthetist. As the potency and side-effects of anaesthetic drugs became more apparent, various ingenious pieces of apparatus designed to regulate concentration were introduced, a trend accelerated by the increasing popularity of nitrous oxide. The forerunner of the modern anaesthetic machine was introduced in 1917 by Henry Boyle, and tracheal intubation in 1920 by Ivan Magill, and the stage was set for the highly complex techniques that hold sway today.

How Anaesthetics Work

It is a source of constant embarrassment to the modern, scientific anaesthetist that we are still in the dark as to the true mode of action of general anaesthetic agents. This is not the place for a detailed explanation of the various theories currently holding sway, but some general points can be made.

A wide range of agents can produce a state of reversible unconsciousness, and it therefore seems likely that there is no specific receptor for these drugs in the central nervous system but that their effect is primarily a physical one. The potency of anaesthetic agents is closely related to their lipid solubility, and this give us an obvious clue towards site of action, which is presumed to be in the cell membrane of the neurone. Somewhat more difficult to work into a common unifying theory of anaesthesia is the unlikely fact that the anaesthetic effect of any agent can be at least partly reversed by submitting the subject to a raised atmospheric pressure. It is generally thought that the mode of action is via swelling of the cell membrane, thus closing channels in the membrane which are responsible for the propagation of the nerve impulse. Certainly, there is no clinical effect upon peripheral nerve fibres at clinical concentrations, so the action probably takes place at synapses or in unmyelinated sections of the axon.

The bottom line is that, although the potency, adverse effects and clinical application of anaesthetic agents are all well documented, we are still rather ignorant of precisely how they actually work.

Balanced Anaesthesia

The modern concept of 'balanced anaesthesia' arises from the understanding that it may be better for the patient if the anaesthetist achieves a 'light' rather than a 'deep' level of anaesthesia. This should not be surprising in itself, as the adverse effects of the powerful anaesthetic agents, discussed later in this chapter and also in Chapter 3, become more apparent as higher doses are used. Light anaesthesia, however, has its own problems – even if awareness is prevented (see below), surgical stimulation will cause catecholamine release, resulting in cardiovascular instability, and the patient may even move during surgery, a particularly upsetting event for all concerned, even though the patient remains blissfully unaware.

Balanced anaesthesia requires the use of other drugs to supplement the anaesthetic, thus preventing the undesirable consequences of light anaesthesia described above. Powerful opioid drugs, such as morphine or fentanyl, are used to provide intense analgesia and dampen the adrenal response to surgical stimulation. Neuromuscular blocking agents ('muscle relaxants') prevent movement of the unconscious patient and provide better access for the surgeon to areas such as the abdominal cavity.

The Airway

Management of the airway is so basic to the practice of good anaesthesia that no apology need be given for covering it in some detail here, particularly as it is a skill that will serve the emergent doctor in whatever field he or she chooses to practise.

Obstruction

During anaesthesia, the soft tissues of the oro-pharynx and the relaxed tongue tend to interfere with the passage of air from mouth to trachea, and it would be a rare event indeed to find a patient who maintained a completely clear airway without assistance while anaesthetized. Even during normal sleep, many of us snore when lying on our backs, and this is the audible result of partial airway obstruction. This effect is greatly magnified during the 'deep sleep' of general anaesthesia, and can often lead to complete airway obstruction, characterized by a 'rocking' movement of the chest and abdomen and a lack of any sound at all from the patient (as air must pass through the pharynx for snoring to occur). Maintenance of a clear airway, therefore, is the first and most important skill learnt by the trainee anaesthetist, and its application rapidly becomes second nature. Failure to maintain an airway, for whatever reason, is the most common cause of death during anaesthesia.

Basic Maintenance (Figure 1.1)

In most patients, an acceptably clear airway can be obtained by the simple expedient of extending the neck and elevating the jaw. This combined manoeuvre has the effect of 'straightening' the route from mouth to trachea and lifting the root of the tongue off the posterior wall of the oro-pharynx.

The most important adjunct to basic airway maintenance is the oral Guedel airway (see Chapter 4) which helps to bring the tongue away from the posterior pharynx, although nasally inserted versions have also become very popular.

Laryngeal Mask Airway

The laryngeal mask airway, now universally abbreviated to LMA, has rapidly achieved prominence as a 'halfway house' between the oral airway and the tracheal tube. By cleverly combining the role of the Guedel airway

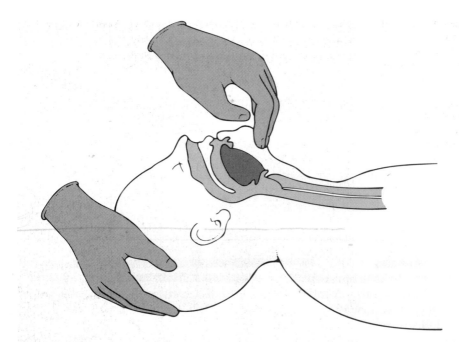

Figure 1.1 Basic airway maintenance using head tilt to extend the neck and chin lift to elevate the jaw.

and the anaesthetic face mask in providing a clear passage and an airtight delivery system for anaesthetic gases, it has freed the anaesthetist's right hand from the patient's face and ushered in a new era of spontaneously breathing anaesthesia (see page 66).

To the uninitiated, the sight of the shaft of an LMA protruding from a patient's mouth invites obvious comparison with a tracheal tube, and this may lead to an unjustified confidence in the patency and protection of the airway. Several incidents reported in recent years in the anaesthetic literature bear witness to the hazards that may result from such an unwarranted assumption. The LMA is a blessing when used within its limitations, but a curse when stretched beyond its intended limits.

Tracheal Intubation

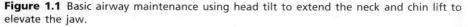

Tracheal intubation remains the only way of guaranteeing /securing an airway in the face of changes of posture and surgical interference, and is also the only way to protect the trachea from soiling by regurgitated stomach contents (see below).

The basic difficulty with tracheal intubation is that, of the two routes that a tube passed into the hypopharynx can take, the tracheal is the one less likely to be followed. Although some anaesthetists have the almost magical talent of being able to blindly pass a nasally directed tube into the trachea 100 per cent of the time, most of us require some help from a laryngoscope.

Figure 1.2 One of the authors demonstrates the ideal head position to facilitate tracheal intubation: Note the flexion of the lower cervical spine and the extension at the atlanto-axial joint.

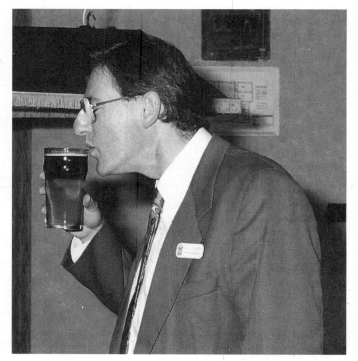

The most commonly used approach to oral tracheal intubation involves putting the head in a position described as 'scenting the morning air' but more familiar to medical students as 'taking the first sip from a full pint of beer' (Figure 1.2). This brings the mouth, oro-pharynx and trachea into as straight a line as possible, thus making it easier to see the tracheal inlet when the laryngoscope is used to elevate the epiglottis (Figure 1.3).

The Difficult Airway

Although airway control /is usually a matter of routine, it can sometimes prove to be extremely difficult. Difficulty may arise as a result of local inflammation, anatomical abnormalities, tumours, cranio-facial syndromes, bleeding, trauma or a multitude of other causes. A difficult airway that is detected before induction of anaesthesia may be a nuisance, but the sudden appreciation of airway problems once unconsciousness has occurred can result in life-threatening consequences. It should be apparent that a careful assessment of the airway is one of the most vital parts of the pre-operative visit, and a variety of tests have been described to predict difficult intubation (Figure 1.4(a) and (b)).

The management of difficult intubation is a complex topic, but the most important principle is that the patient is not at risk until anaesthesia has been induced. It therefore follows that the safest route is to secure the airway by

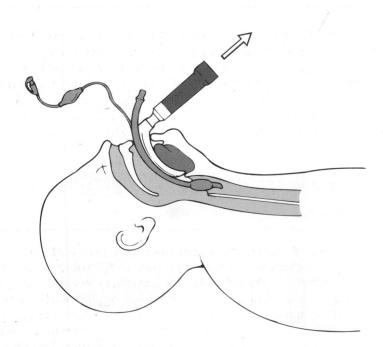

Figure 1.3 Tracheal intubation using the Macintosh laryngoscope.

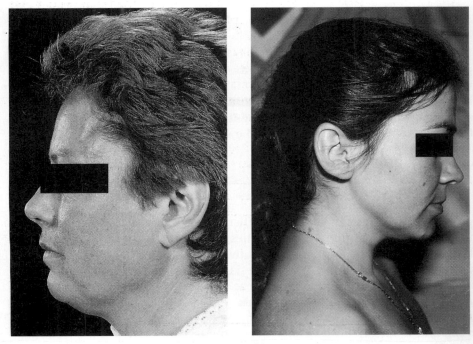

(a)   (b)

Figure 1.4 (a) A profile heralding a difficult airway. Note the receding chin and short neck. (b) An easy-looking airway, but this girl's juvenile rheumatoid arthritis has restricted her neck and jaw movements and intubation is very difficult.

intubation while the patient is awake. Various techniques have been described for awake intubation, but one accepted method is to produce anaesthesia of the airway by topical application of local anaesthetic agents, passing a fibreoptic scope into the trachea, and then 'railroading' a tracheal tube over the scope. In skilled hands, awake intubation does not need to be any more traumatic than venepuncture, and learning the use of the fibreoptic scope is an important part of the modern anaesthetist's training.

Other Hazards

Gastric Contents

Apart from loss of airway patency, an unconscious patient is at risk of regurgitating stomach contents which may then pass down the trachea into the lungs. We are normally protected from this unsavoury event by the powerful gag and cough reflexes that defend the trachea against such soiling, but these disappear at quite light levels of anaesthesia. Fortunately, gastric contents are not free to empty upwards into the oesophagus at will; the gastro-oesophageal junction incorporates a sphincter mechanism that must be overcome before regurgitation occurs.

The effect of aspiration of gastric contents upon the lungs is dependent on several factors, chief of which is the pH of the aspirate. The cut-off point appears to be in the region of pH 2.5. Above this level, aspiration causes relatively mild bronchial and alveolar inflammation, sometimes with superadded infection: below pH 2.5 progressive pulmonary fibrosis occurs, leading to deterioration of lung function and adult respiratory distress syndrome (ARDS), a complication with a high mortality rate. Volume also appears, not surprisingly, to play a part – a low volume of aspirated material causes less damage than a high volume, and the widely quoted, but experimentally shaky, cut-off point is 0.4 mL/kg body weight.

In the field of obstetric anaesthesia, where the delay in gastric emptying imposed by labour, the high intragastric pressures caused by the gravid uterus, and the occasional necessity for emergency general anaesthesia combine to produce a high incidence of aspiration, the condition is known as Mendelson's syndrome, after the North American obstetrician who first described the incidence and causes of the problem. Mendelson's syndrome is on the decrease (see below), but until recently was one of the most common causes of maternal death in the UK.

Fasting

The pre-operative period of fasting is one thing that all surgical patients remember about their hospital stay, and it is hard to imagine a surgical ward without the festoons of 'nil by mouth' signs around the beds. The purpose of the pre-operative fast is to reduce the volume of gastric contents, thus making them safer; the reduction in volume also lowers intragastric pressure, so making regurgitation less likely. Fasting periods are gradually getting shorter as our understanding of gastric physiology progresses, and many hospitals now employ a '4 hours for solids, 3 hours for liquids' rule.

Despite these precautions, there is plenty of evidence to suggest that a substantial number of elective patients arrive in the anaesthetic room with 'unsafe' stomach contents; we are probably more reliant on the gastro-oesophageal sphincter mechanism than we would like to believe.

HIGH-RISK PATIENTS

In some groups of patients (Table 1.1) it is not enough to rely on fasting, and two other approaches may be taken. Pharmacological methods may be used to ensure safe gastric pH and volume, and mechanical precautions can be employed to protect the trachea from regurgitated material.

Drug therapy usually consists of a combination of histamine-2 receptor antagonists (cimetidine, ranitidine) to prevent acid production, antacid buffers (sodium citrate) to neutralize any acid already present in the stomach, and drugs to aid gastric emptying (metoclopramide, cisapride). Use of this sort of regimen is seen at its best on the labour suite, where careful attention to detail has probably been responsible for the recent dramatic fall in the incidence of Mendelson's syndrome.

Patients who are particularly at risk, e.g. obstetric patients, trauma victims and those with an acute abdomen, are regarded as having 'dangerous' gastric contents whatever therapy they may have received. In these patients, the trachea is protected by occluding the oesophagus by means of firm pressure on the cricoid cartilage (Sellick's manoeuvre). This pressure is applied just before anaesthesia is induced, and is maintained until the cuff of a properly sited tracheal tube has been inflated, so providing complete protection for the trachea. In combination with a period of pre-induction 100 per cent oxygen (pre-oxygenation) to increase the reserves of oxygen in the lungs in case of difficulty with the airway and the use of a fast-acting neuro-muscular blocker such as suxamethonium (to facilitate rapid tracheal intuba-tion), the process is known as 'rapid-sequence induction'.

It is often forgotten that these patients are equally at risk of aspiration at the end of an operation, and that this is best prevented by not removing the

Table 1.1 Conditions predisposing to regurgitation and pulmonary aspiration of gastric contents

Pregnancy after 20 weeks' gestation
Trauma victims who eat four hours or less before their accident
Acute abdomen
Gastric reflux due to hiatus hernia
Hypersecretion of gastric acid
Use of drugs which slow gastric emptying, especially opioids

tracheal tube until protective reflexes have returned, and by careful monitoring in a post-operative recovery area.

Respiratory Depression

All modern, centrally acting anaesthetic drugs, whether intravenous or inhalational, cause a degree of respiratory depression, and this can be dangerous if unrecognized, especially in combination with a degree of respiratory obstruction. The situation can be further worsened by the concomitant administration of other respiratory-depressant drugs, such as opioids. The two resulting hazards of hypoxaemia (low arterial partial pressure of oxygen) and hypercapnia (raised arterial partial pressure of carbon dioxide) are never far from the mind of the anaesthetist.

Hypoxaemia during general anaesthesia (easily detected with the pulse oximeter) may result from a variety of causes (Table 1.2) but can generally be prevented by the simple expedient of giving a gas mixture with an oxygen concentration of 30 per cent or greater (compared with our usual source of inspired gas, air, which contains 21 per cent). This ploy will, of course, be to no avail if the gas mixture is not getting to the lungs, as in a case of oesophageal intubation, total respiratory obstruction, or disconnection of the breathing/ventilator systems!

Hypercapnia is less easy to control but, in most circumstances, is not hazardous to the patient. As the arterial carbon dioxide tension is inversely proportional to the minute alveolar ventilation, it can be readily seen that hypercapnia inevitably results whenever respiratory depression occurs. Anaesthetists monitor arterial carbon dioxide by measuring the end-tidal concentration of the gas (the concentration in the last gas to leave the lungs during expiration), generally quite a close approximation. We normally maintain our end-tidal carbon dioxide partial pressure at around 5–5.5 kPa, but values as high as 7 kPa may be seen during anaesthesia when the patient is breathing spontaneously. Levels in this range may cause peripheral vasodilatation and a slight increase in cardiac output. Higher levels run the risk of causing CNS depression, which lowers the minute volume further and can trigger a vicious cycle of carbon dioxide retention. Fortunately, we

Table 1.2 Causes of hypoxaemia during general anaesthesia

Hypoxic gas mixture
Central respiratory depression
Respiratory obstruction
Disconnection of breathing system
Pneumothorax
Ventilation–perfusion mismatch caused by:
   Hypotension
   Positive-pressure ventilation
   Positioning of patients in prone or lateral positions

can control this at any time by simply taking over the patient's respiration and commencing positive-pressure ventilation, using high minute volumes to 'blow-off' excessive carbon dioxide.

Cardiovascular Depression

Most anaesthetic agents lower blood pressure, either by reducing cardiac output, by causing vasodilatation or by a combination of the two. Ether was a proud exception, of historical interest only now, and ketamine has the reputation of maintaining, or even raising, blood pressure in the compromised patient.

It is not uncommon to see systolic blood pressures below 90 mmHg after induction, especially before the surgical stimulus is applied. Newcomers to the field are often surprised at how sanguine the anaesthetist remains in the face of what would be regarded as a 'dangerously' low blood pressure in an awake patient, and student nurses have been heard to comment adversely on the cavalier attitude of the man at the top of the table. The fact is that hypotension of this order is very well tolerated when drug-induced (and therefore largely due to vasodilatation) whereas, if caused by hypovolaemia or cardiogenic shock, it would be far more dangerous. Autoregulation of blood flow to vital organs such as the kidneys and brain seems to be well maintained under anaesthesia in the face of low blood pressure. Hypotension resulting from vasodilatation responds very well to a rapid intravenous infusion of fluid, and specific vasoconstrictors, such as ephedrine, can be used to achieve a faster response if needed. Myocardial depression is often countered by the catecholamine-releasing effect of surgical incision, and inotropic drugs are very rarely required.

Damage to the Peripheries

As well as the central protective reflexes already mentioned, the unconscious patient loses the ability to protect himself from harm in other ways. Noxious peripheral stimuli such as pressure and heat, from which the conscious patient would withdraw, can be inadvertently applied to the anaesthetized subject, and can lead to physical damage.

Correct positioning is an important part of the anaesthetist's care of the patient. All peripheries must be padded and protected from interference by the surgeon and his henchmen. No part of the body should come into contact with any metallic fixture, thus preventing the risk of skin burns due to diathermy current finding an alternative pathway to earth. When positions other than the standard supine posture are required, particular care must be taken to avoid unnecessary strain on pressure areas, joints and nerves.

Nerves can be damaged by pressure from external sources such as poles and supports. Particular attention must be paid to poorly protected nerves situated close to the skin – the classic examples are the ulnar nerve at the elbow and the common peroneal nerve as it passes over the head of the fibula. Damage to nerves can also be caused by overstretching due to poor positioning; the brachial plexus, for example, can be affected if the shoulder is abducted to more than 90°, particularly if the head is turned away from the extended arm.

Skin can be damaged as a direct result of pressure, especially when perfusion is poor or skin is fragile (elderly, hypotension, steroid treatment). Patients undergoing very prolonged surgery are particularly prone to skin damage, and care must be taken to pad pressure areas as much as possible and to prevent shear stresses which will greatly speed up the damage.

Eyes must be protected carefully to prevent corneal abrasions from surgical drapes or small particles getting onto the conjunctiva. Many anaesthetists now cover the eye with a protective gel and then tape it closed. Even more dangerous is the effect of pressure when the patient is prone. If the eyes rest directly on the table, thus bearing the full weight of the patient's head, considerable pressure is placed on the retina; this can cause blindness, and great care must therefore be taken to ensure that the weight of the head is supported on the forehead or side of the face.

Awareness

Should an anaesthetic become too light, as a result of either operator error or a particularly 'resistant' patient, it is possible that the patient may regain a degree of consciousness, commonly referred to as anaesthetic awareness, during the operation. This may range from a muddled appreciation of conversation in the theatre, through a painless memory of physical sensation, right up to the (fortunately rare) nightmare scenario of total consciousness, full pain appreciation and complete post-operative recall. Of course, any patient retaining the ability to move would quickly bring the situation to the attention of the theatre team; the real problem occurs for the patient who is aware but unable to move due to the effect of neuromuscular blocking agents. Needless to say, patients in this unimaginable position are severely traumatized by the events, and considerable damages have been awarded in Court in such cases.

Surprisingly, some slight degree of awareness may occur in up to 1 per cent of cases; most of these go unreported because the patient does not remember what happened, a phenomenon known as retrograde amnesia. Full awareness is very uncommon but is particularly associated with Caesarean section (because light anaesthesia is used to avoid neonatal sedation) and cardiac surgery (because the potent anaesthetic agents are often avoided due to their effects on the cardiovascular system).

It is a considerable failing on the part of our specialty that no reliable monitor yet exists to measure depth of anaesthesia – although, in mitigation, it is not for want of trying. The best method to detect awareness in the paralysed patient is probably careful use of clinical signs such as blood pressure, pulse rate and sweating: the best way to prevent it is by sensible use of potent volatile agents and powerful analgesics.

Homeostasis

As well as maintaining anaesthesia, one of the anaesthetist's tasks is to ensure that, as far as possible, the patient leaves the operating theatre in as healthy a state as possible. Surgery damages tissues, causes bleeding and results in pain, but there are other, more subtle effects that need to be borne in mind.

Fluid Replacement

The average adult patient needs about 2 mL/kg per h of fluid to maintain a normal fluid balance, and during surgery this is usually provided as a balanced salt solution such as Compound Sodium Lactate (Hartmann's solution); frequently, however, fluid requirements can be much greater than this. Exposure of warm, moist body cavities to the cold, dry atmosphere of the operating theatre (e.g. during laparotomy or thoracotomy) can result in considerable 'invisible' fluid loss by evaporation and convection. This can be exacerbated by relocation of extracellular fluid into tissues such as the peritoneum during handling of the bowel or omentum – the so-called 'third space' loss. Even without significant blood loss, this can result in baseline intraoperative fluid requirement being as high as 10 mL/kg per h (700 mL per h in a normal adult male). This would usually be replaced with a crystal-loid fluid such as Hartmann's solution, but some practitioners prefer smaller volumes of a colloid such as gelatin or starch solutions – controversies about the correct approach have been raging for many years and provide useful employment for itinerant anaesthetic lecturers.

Blood loss is usually well tolerated up to around 10–15 per cent of total blood volume. After this, a colloid solution is usually used to boost the intravascular volume, and blood transfusion should be considered when blood loss exceeds 20 per cent of blood volume.

Temperature

Operating theatres need to be kept at a relatively high temperature if signifi-cant hypothermia is to be prevented, and this is often impracticable if the environment is to be tolerable to the operating team, who are working fully clad under bright lights. Heat loss can be a particular problem with very young patients, who have a high surface area to volume ratio and therefore lose heat quickly, and very old patients, who often have little fat to insulate them. Major, prolonged surgery, especially involving open body cavities, can also exacerbate heat loss and every effort should be made by the anaesthetist to maintain the patient's temperature. Hot air or water blankets may be used on the operating table, and intravenous fluid is often warmed before infusion. The anaesthetic gases may be warmed and humidified, as the airways and lungs are an important site for heat loss, and the patient should be covered as much as possible, with the obvious exception of the operation site. Even with these precautions, core temperature may drop during a long procedure, and continuous temperature monitoring, often rectally or via the oesophagus, should be employed.

Conduct of a General Anaesthetic

To give an idea of the practical aspects of general anaesthesia, this next section briefly goes through the processes involved in anaesthetizing a healthy man in his 20s for hernia repair. The scenario assumes the use a laryngeal mask airway and spontaneous respiration, but there are as many alternatives as there are anaesthetists (and probably more)!

Induction

Following a pre-operative visit by the anaesthetist, a 4-hour period of fasting, and an oral premedication of temazepam 20 mg, the patient arrives in the anaesthetic room, drowsy but awake. The anaesthetic assistant places ECG electrodes on the patient's chest and connects ECG, automatic blood pressure monitor and oximeter. The anaesthetist inserts a small intravenous cannula into a vein on the back of the hand (after judicious infiltration of lignocaine), and gives the patient 100 per cent oxygen to breathe from the anaesthetic machine, checking this with an oxygen analyser.

After testing the correct placement of the cannula, the anaesthetist gives morphine 3 mg, then administers propofol slowly until the patient closes his eyes. After taking the anaesthetic mask from her assistant, the anaesthetist reduces the oxygen from 8 to 2 L per minute, starts nitrous oxide 4 L per minute and gradually introduces enflurane from the vapourizer until 3 per cent is reached. After breathing this mixture for 2 minutes, the patient's pupils are central and mid-constricted. Our anaesthetist then temporarily turns off the anaesthetic agents (to prevent pollution of the anaesthetic room), removes the mask, takes the LMA and inserts it with a single smooth movement until it comes to rest over the laryngeal inlet. The assistant inflates the cuff and tapes the LMA to the face while the breathing system is reconnected. After confirming that there is no respiratory obstruction, the anaesthetist tapes the eyes, disconnects the monitors and moves the patient into theatre, where he is carefully lifted onto the operating table and positioned for surgery.

Maintenance

Monitors are connected as in the anaesthetic room, but with the addition of a multi-gas analyser (carbon dioxide, oxygen, nitrous oxide and volatile agent) attached to the end of the LMA. Enflurane is continued at 1.5–3 per cent throughout surgery, and further small boluses of morphine given, the total dose being 10 mg. Blood pressure, heart rate, ECG, oxygen saturation and end-tidal carbon dioxide are monitored continuously and charted at 5-minute intervals throughout the procedure, and post-operative analgesia and anti-emetics prescribed. At the end of the operation, the surgeon injects bupivacaine around the wound at the request of the anaesthetist and administers a diclofenac suppository, for longer-term analgesia.

Recovery

As the last few sutures are tied, the anaesthetist switches off the enflurane and nitrous oxide, running 100 per cent oxygen at 6 L per minute. After confirming acceptable oxygen saturation and cardiovascular parameters, she and the assistant lift the patient on to a trolley and turn him onto his side – oxygen is administered via a 'T-piece' apparatus.

As they enter the recovery area, the patient opens his eyes and moves his hands towards the LMA. The recovery nurse deflates the cuff, removes the LMA and starts oxygen by mask. Oxygen saturation and blood pressure are again measured. After 20 minutes, the patient is returned to the surgical ward fully orientated, comfortable and not feeling sick. The anaesthetist then retires gracefully for a cup of coffee.

The Recovery Unit

The role of the recovery unit is an important one, and it would be unusual for a patient in the UK nowadays not to stop, however briefly, in this area before transfer to the ward.

Even with the use of modern anaesthetic agents, it would be asking too much to expect a patient to reverse magically from a state of surgical anaesthesia to fully awake in a few seconds, and the recovery unit provides an intermediate care area where the patient can be nursed on a one-to-one basis while he recovers his protective airway reflexes and regains consciousness. Recovery nurses are trained specifically in the care of the unconscious patient and are often doubly qualified so that they can assist the anaesthetist in theatre.

While in recovery, the patient's vital signs are monitored frequently, dressings checked for bleeding, and regular observations of fluid input and output established. One of the most important roles of the recovery nurse, however, is the control of post-operative pain. Techniques for this may range from simply helping the patient to find a comfortable position, through the setting up of patient-controlled analgesia or an epidural infusion, to the administration of intravenous boluses of opioids. This topic is covered in more detail in Chapter 7.

Anaesthesia for Children and the Elderly

Some specific aspects of anaesthesia at the extremes of life are listed in Table 1.3.

Table 1.3 Points to consider in small children and old patients

Very young patients	Old patients
Co-operation	Delicate skin and veins
Difficult venous access	Concurrent disease
Excessive salivation	Concomitant medication
Intubation more difficult	Decreased renal and hepatic function
Risk of tracheal ischaemia from tube	Care with pressure areas
More rapid oxygen desaturation	Sensitive to anaesthetic drugs
Resistance to anaesthetic drugs	Prone to cardiorespiratory embarrassment
Greater fluid requirements for weight	Less tolerant of fluid loss or overload
Low blood volume	Post-operative confusion
Difficult parents!	

Some Current Controversies

Many anaesthetists feel that too many operations are performed under general anaesthesia in the UK. Certainly, in the rest of Europe, particularly Scandinavia and the Netherlands, regional anaesthesia is used far more commonly.

The advent of the laryngeal mask airway has reopened the debate over the relative benefits of spontaneously breathing anaesthesia and anaesthesia aided by neuromuscular blockade and intermittent positive-pressure ventilation (IPPV).

The introduction of truly short-acting intravenous agents (e.g. propofol) has meant that anaesthetists can re-examine the practice of using volatile agents for maintenance. The possibility of total intravenous anaesthesia (TIVA), achieved by using a continuous propofol infusion, is now a realistic alternative to more conventional techniques (Figure 1.5).

The pros and cons of these arguments are considered in Table 1.4.

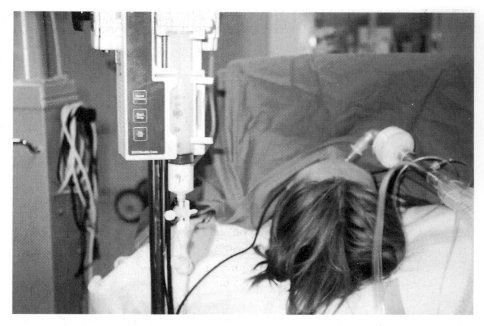

Figure 1.5 Maintenance of anaesthesia by a continuous intravenous infusion of propofol.

Table 1.4 Some anaesthetic controversies

General anaesthesia versus regional anaesthesia	
General	*Regional*
Easier to achieve acceptable result	Less 'sledgehammer' approach
Expected by a lot of patients	Safer intraoperatively
More relaxed atmosphere in theatre	Probably fewer post-operative problems
Wider applicability	Encourages more delicate surgery
Quicker	Patient involvement, e.g. Caesarean section
Spontaneous respiration versus IPPV	
Spontaneous	*IPPV*
Safer if disconnection occurs	Lighter anaesthesia
More 'physiological'	Better muscle relaxation
Better assessment of anaesthetic depth	Prevention of hypercapnia
Minimal risk of awareness	Safer if large doses of opioids are required
Maintenance with volatile agent versus total intravenous anaesthesia (TIVA)	
Volatile	*TIVA*
Better assessment of anaesthetic depth	No atmospheric pollution
Better control over blood pressure	Less post-operative 'hangover'
More familiar technique	Single drug for induction and maintenance
Less reliance on technology	Possible lower incidence of nausea
Cheaper	

Key Points

- The exact mode of action of general anaesthetic agents is unknown.

- 'Balanced anaesthesia' is a combination of sleep, analgesia and muscle relaxation.

- Airway maintenance is the most important task of the anaesthetist during general anaesthesia.

- Tracheal intubation is the only way to guarantee a clear airway and protect the lungs from aspiration of gastric contents.

- The laryngeal mask airway (LMA) is an important adjunct to airway maintenance, but should not be considered as a substitute for tracheal intubation.

- The anaesthetist is responsible for positioning the patient and ensuring that vulnerable areas are protected from pressure.

- Constant vigilance is essential during maintenance of even the most minor anaesthetic to prevent hypoxia, respiratory and cardiovascular depression and awareness.

- A good recovery unit is essential to enable a smooth transition from the anaesthetized state to a safe level of consciousness and comfort.

Further Reading

Aitkenhead, A.R., Smith, G. 1996: *Textbook of anaesthesia* (3rd edn). Edinburgh: Churchill Livingstone.

Atkinson, R.S., Rushman, G.B., Lee, J.A. 1987: *A synopsis of anaesthesia* (10th edn). Bristol: Wright.

2 Local and Regional Anaesthesia

Introduction

There is a shift in current practice away from general anaesthesia, and towards techniques using local anaesthetic drugs. Britain has not moved as fast as other European countries in this respect, but the trend is obvious. The change in emphasis can be illustrated by comparing the mottos of the Association of Anaesthetists of Great Britain and Ireland, founded 1935 ('In Somno Securitas' – safety in sleep), and the Royal College of Anaesthetists, founded 1989 ('Divinum Sedare Dolorem' – it is good to relieve pain). Most anaesthetists would choose a regional technique, where possible, if they ever needed surgery, and in some fields, notably obstetrics, urology and orthopaedics, some form of regional block is rapidly becoming the norm.

A word about terminology is applicable here. The term 'local' normally means the use of a drug to produce anaesthesia by topical application, infiltration or ring block. 'Regional' is a term reserved to describe major nerve blocks or spinal/epidural techniques. However the terms are often used interchangeably and, because both approaches use the same group of drugs and have their effects by blocking nerve conduction, there are more similarities than differences between them.

The advantages and disadvantages of regional compared to general anaesthesia are summarized in Table 2.1. Safe and effective use of regional techniques obviously requires a good working knowledge of the available drugs – this is discussed in Chapter 3. A calm anaesthetist with an understanding of the local anatomy, a gentle surgeon, and a confident, well-prepared patient are all important factors in the success of a regional block.

Each local anaesthetic technique has its hazards and pitfalls (Table 2.2), but some general principles should always be considered when using these drugs. In particular, a history of allergy to local anaesthetics must be sought; most of the currently used drugs are amides, and sensitivity to one, although rare, can mean a major anaphylactic response to any of this group of drugs. This, in conjunction with the adverse cardiovascular and neurological effects of local anaesthetic overdosage, means that equipment for cardiopulmonary resuscitation must be immediately available when local anaesthetic drugs are used. Furthermore, when large doses or 'high-tech' blocks are being used

Table 2.1 Regional versus general anaesthesia

Advantages	Disadvantages

Avoids adverse effects of general anaesthetic agents:
  Respiratory depression
  Cardiovascular depression
  Nausea/vomiting
  'Hangover'
	Toxicity of local anaesthetic drugs (see Table 2.2)

Avoids potential hazards of unconsciousness:
  Loss of airway
  Aspiration of gastric contents
  Damage to joints, skin, etc.
  through malpositioning
	Often difficult techniques:
	  More risk of failure or partial success
	  More discomfort while performing block
	  May take longer to establish
	  anaesthesia, so delaying operating list

Minimizes endocrine stress response to surgery Decreased post-operative pain Earlier discharge from hospital	Greater co-operation needed from patient Sets time limit for surgery Restricts flexibility of surgeon if operation needs to be more extensive

Table 2.2 Hazards of local anaesthetic agents

Local administration

  Inadvertent intravascular injection—rapid onset of toxic effects
  Inadvertent intraneuronal injection—nerve damage
  Incorrect use of adrenaline-containing solution—tissue necrosis
  Vasodilatation—increased bleeding
  Tachyphylaxis—reduced effectiveness of repeated doses
  Spread of infection—if injected into infected area

Regional anaesthesia

  Marked vasodilatation—fall in blood pressure
  Major nerve compression—haematoma or abscess formation
  Large doses may be needed—risk of overdosage

Effects of overdose

  Cardiovascular system   Bradycardia
                                Fall in cardiac contractility → hypotension
                                Cardiac arrest

NB. Cocaine and adrenaline-containing solutions cause tachycardia and hypertension

  Central nervous system   Paraesthesiae, especially around mouth
                                 Anxiety
                                 Tremors
                                 Fitting
                                 Coma

(intravenous regional anaesthesia, major nerve blocks, epidural and spinal anaesthesia), the patient should be fully fasted – aspiration of gastric contents remains one of the most common causes of death following regional anaesthesia. Automated monitoring of vital functions – ECG, blood pressure and arterial oxygen saturation – is also mandatory in these cases. In addition, an intravenous cannula must always be inserted before the block is performed in case emergency drugs or fluids are required. In short, the same precautions should be taken as for a general anaesthetic.

Regional anaesthesia should not be thought of as a universal solution to the management of sick patients needing surgery. The vasodilatation that routinely accompanies spinal or epidural anaesthesia can be very hazardous for the shocked patient, and is discussed further later in this chapter. In cases of respiratory or cardiovascular disease, the control of airway and oxygenation afforded by tracheal intubation may well make general anaesthesia the safer option.

This chapter will go on to discuss the use of local anaesthesia, from the humble but important technique of local infiltration to the *pièce de résistance* of the spinal block.

Topical Anaesthesia

Local anaesthetic drugs readily penetrate mucous membranes, and this route is frequently used in clinical practice. The simple lozenge used to relieve a sore throat (usually containing benzocaine or amethocaine) is a case in point, and other sites in which this technique is used include the conjunctiva, nasal mucosa and urethra, usually before examination or instrumentation.

Although regarded as very safe, drugs are absorbed so rapidly across mucous membranes that serum concentration of the local anaesthetic rises almost as rapidly as when given intravenously. Toxic blood levels can therefore be achieved surprisingly easily. This is of especial relevance to the ENT surgeon, who uses cocaine to anaesthetize the nasal mucosa. Cocaine is particularly useful because, alone among the local anaesthetics, it has vasoconstrictor properties, thus causing the mucosa to shrink down and making bleeding less likely – very helpful during examination. However, the toxic dose of a 20 per cent solution of cocaine when applied topically is 3 mg/kg – a 70 kg man would be limited to just over 1 mL (see Table 2.3). This is, of course, assuming that he is healthy; cocaine potentiates the action of adrenaline, causing hypertension and tachycardia, and should not be used in patients with poorly controlled hypertension or ischaemic heart disease. It can readily be seen that topical anaesthesia is not as harmless as often thought.

Until recently, effective skin anaesthesia could not be achieved without injection. The development of a lignocaine–prilocaine cream (EMLA – eutectic mixture of local anaesthetics) means that topical anaesthesia of intact skin is now possible, although the cream must be applied at least one hour in advance and covered with an occlusive dressing if it is to be effective. EMLA

Table 2.3 Maximum recommended doses of local anaesthetic agents

Lignocaine alone	3 mg/kg
Lignocaine with adrenaline	7 mg/kg
Bupivacaine	2 mg/kg
Prilocaine	6 mg/kg
Cocaine	3 mg/kg

1% solution contains 10 mg/mL
1:1000 solution ≡ 0.1% ≡ 1 mg/mL

is particularly valuable in paediatric practice, where it has done much to alleviate fear of venepuncture and other injections, and its use in allowing pain-free intravenous induction of anaesthesia has reduced the stress for patient and anaesthetist alike.

Local anaesthetic drugs are not the only way to produce skin anaesthesia. Extreme cold, usually produced by using an ethyl chloride spray, was popular for paediatric venepuncture and abscess incision before EMLA was introduced. The technique was rarely 100 per cent effective, however, and had the disadvantage of causing cold-induced vasoconstriction just when a really good vein was needed!

Infiltration

Probably the most common use of local anaesthetic drugs is for infiltration of the tissues around a wound in the accident and emergency department, or before excision of a skin lesion in minor surgery. Anaesthesia of quite large areas can be achieved in minutes, and the method can be used successfully and safely by anyone who has taken note of a few important points.

Choice of Drug

Lignocaine is widely preferred, but care should be taken to use the lowest available concentration (0.5 per cent). Stronger solutions only provide an advantage when large nerves are to be blocked, and their inappropriate use makes toxicity more likely. Adrenaline-containing solutions are often chosen as they cause local vasoconstriction, thus reducing bleeding and minimizing systemic absorption of the local anaesthetic: when using adrenaline care should be taken in patients with cardiovascular disease. Adrenaline-containing solutions must be strictly avoided in areas containing small end-arteries such as the digits – vasoconstriction around the base of an extremity supplied by an end-artery acts like an irreversible pharmacological tourniquet, and ischaemia followed by gangrene has led to loss of toes and fingers in the past, and will doubtless do so again.

Prevention of Intravascular Injection

Whenever the needle tip is moved, always pull back on the syringe plunger before injection to confirm that blood cannot be aspirated. Inadvertent intravascular injection means that the block will not work and, more importantly, that systemic toxicity is much more likely.

Ring Block

This is a quick, effective method for anaesthetizing an extremity, typically a finger or toe. Useful in accident and emergency prior to toilet and suturing of wounds, a ring block involves infiltrating local anaesthetic subcutaneously around the full circumference of the extremity proximal to the operation site. In practice, ring block is often combined with a specific nerve block, e.g. digital nerves for the finger. Combinations of ring and nerve blocks can also be used more proximally at the wrist or ankle for hand or foot surgery.

Nerve Blocks

It has been said that every nerve is accessible to the skilled anaesthetist; this may be so, but some are more easily found than others, and only the more common blocks are shown in Figure 2.1(a) and (b).

A good knowledge of anatomy is essential when performing a nerve block, particularly as nerves have a distressing habit of running close to major blood vessels; careful aspiration of the syringe before injecting is therefore particularly vital. Accurate nerve location is important for a successful block and, as well as relying on anatomical landmarks, the prudent anaesthetist may try to elicit paraesthesia in the relevant area with his needle tip, or even use a low-current nerve stimulator. This device uses a small electric current which causes muscle twitching when the tip of the needle is close to a nerve. Obviously, the nerve stimulator is only of use when seeking a nerve with motor as well as sensory functions.

The local anaesthetic agent used depends upon the procedure being contemplated. If a large nerve is being blocked, a concentrated solution should be used, e.g. 1 per cent or even 2 per cent lignocaine, and a longer acting drug such as bupivacaine should be considered if prolonged surgery is planned. Etidocaine is very effective at penetrating large nerves, but sometimes produces a better motor than sensory block. Since local anaesthetic drugs are more effective in a neutral or slightly alkaline environment, carbonated lignocaine (with added bicarbonate) has been used to improve the quality of block of large nerves, such as the sciatic. When using large volumes of concentrated agents, the maximum safe dose must always be borne in mind (see Table 2.3). This is particularly important when several nerve blocks are being performed at once, e.g. sciatic, femoral, obturator and lateral cutaneous nerve of the thigh for a complete leg block.

Of the techniques shown in Figure 2.1(a) and (b), femoral nerve block deserves a particular mention. Easy and quick to perform, it is especially useful in casualty to ease the pain of a fractured femoral shaft. Multiple intercostal blocks can be of great benefit to patients with fractured ribs, but the proximity of the parietal pleura to the intended target must be borne in mind, and a watchful eye kept on the total volume of drug administered to avoid giving a toxic dose. Over-enthusiastic needling can, and often does, cause a pneumothorax, so the wise practitioner will only ever attempt an intercostal block on one side of the chest, and will always take a post-block chest X-ray. The brachial plexus is accessible by any one of three routes (Figure 2.2), the axillary approach probably being the safest, but the interscalene route affording a better block of the upper arm, important if a surgical tourniquet is to be used. Brachial plexus blocks are performed more frequently than leg blocks, largely because epidural or spinal anaesthesia is a simpler route when leg surgery is planned.

As with all local anaesthesia, the usefulness of nerve blocks is limited by the duration of action of the drug used. Some nerves, however, are sheathed in discrete neurovascular bundles, along which a flexible catheter can be passed after insertion through a needle. This can be 'topped-up' at intervals in the manner of an epidural block (see below), allowing for prolonged surgery. Continuous brachial plexus block is the most common example of this technique, and many an anaesthetist has spent a long night topping-up a brachial plexus catheter while the plastic surgeons painstakingly re-attach a couple of severed fingers! The block can also be extended into the post-operative period to provide pain relief.

Intravenous Regional Anaesthesia

IVRA, or Bier's block, is used to anaesthetize the arm (or less commonly, the leg), classically before reduction of a fractured wrist, but also for minor surgery such as relief of carpal tunnel syndrome. After inserting an intravenous cannula (usually in the dorsum of the hand), the limb is exsanguinated by elevation or compression, and an occlusive tourniquet inflated on the upper arm. The now isolated and empty vasculature of the arm is filled with a dilute solution of local anaesthetic via the cannula. Prilocaine is the drug of choice for this block, as it offers the best therapeutic ratio between effective and cardiotoxic doses (see below). Surgery can begin after 3–5 minutes, and the tourniquet can be deflated after a period of not less than 20 minutes, by which time most of the drug has been bound to tissues in the arm, and so does not enter the general circulation.

IVRA is so easy and effective that it has gained particular popularity in the accident and emergency department where, in its heyday, long queues of old ladies with Colles' fractures could be found, tourniqueted arms pale

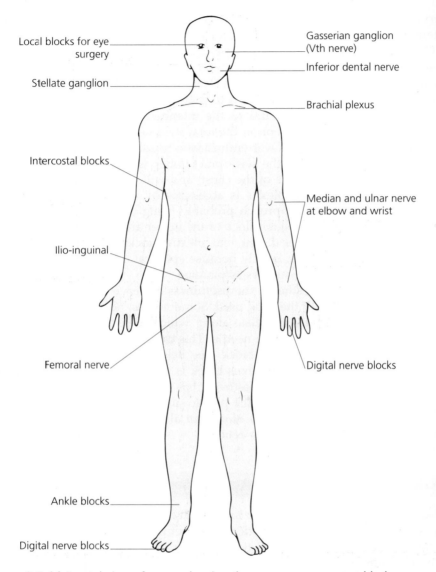

Figure 2.1 (a) Frontal view of a man showing the more common nerve blocks.

and blotchy, waiting for the SHO to come down the line, snap the wrist back into place, apply a backslab plaster, order a check X-ray and send them on their way. Unfortunately, it was not sufficiently widely recognized that the tourniquet was the only barrier between a lethal overdose of local anaesthetic and the heart, and several deaths due to tourniquet (or doctor) failure led to more stringent control of this technique. It should now be mandatory to make sure that the patient is fasted, to have a cannula also in the non-anaesthetized arm for intravenous access, and for someone to be present whose sole job is to look after the tourniquet. With these caveats,

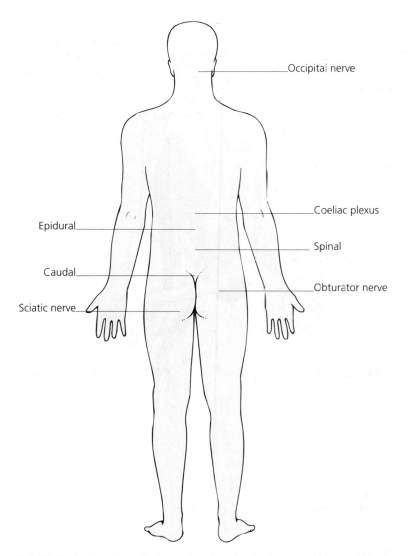

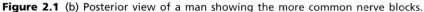

Figure 2.1 (b) Posterior view of a man showing the more common nerve blocks.

however, IVRA remains the quickest and easiest way to achieve regional anaesthesia of a limb.

Spinal and Epidural Anaesthesia

These techniques are really in a separate league to the blocks described above. Although different in execution, effect and application, spinal and epidural anaesthesia have many similarities which will be discussed before going on to further details of the individual methods.

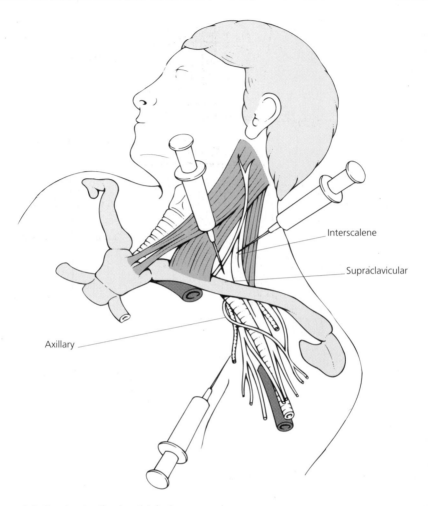

Figure 2.2 Routes to the brachial plexus.

Anatomy (see Figure 2.3)

Afferent sensory nerve fibres enter the spinal cord throughout its length via the dorsal horn. In doing so, they cross the epidural and subarachnoid spaces, where they are vulnerable to block by local anaesthetic drugs. Both of these spaces are usually reached by inserting a needle in the midline between the spinous processes of two vertebrae.

The epidural space is the more superficial, and is reached by passing a needle through the ligamentum flavum, the end-point being identified by loss of resistance to injection of air or saline. Deep to the ligamentum flavum by only a few millimetres, and marking the distal boundary of the epidural space, is the dura mater, with the arachnoid firmly attached. Passage through the dura is marked by a sudden flow of cerebrospinal fluid (CSF) through

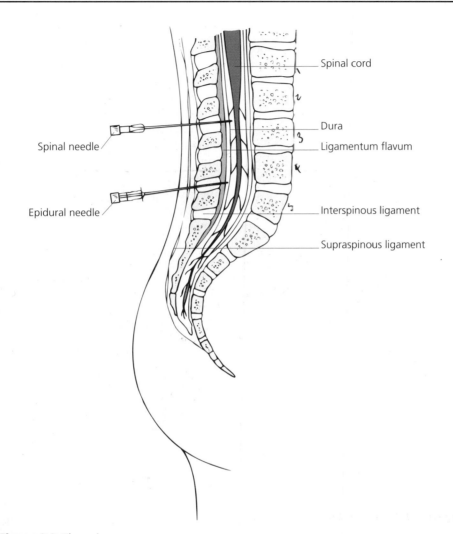

Spinal cord

Dura

Ligamentum flavum

Spinal needle

Epidural needle

Interspinous ligament

Supraspinous ligament

Figure 2.3 The spine.

the needle indicating entry into the subarachnoid space, the target of spinal anaesthesia. The spinal cord terminates at the level of the first lumbar vertebra (second in children) and the floating fronds of the cauda equina tend to move away from a needle tip – for this reason, spinal anaesthesia is performed below this level. Epidural puncture may be performed at any point along the vertebral column, but becomes technically more difficult when straying beyond the lumbosacral region.

Effects of Spinal/Epidural Block

The introduction of local anaesthetic drugs into the epidural or subarachnoid spaces has similar effects, although different in intensity and time scale.

AUTONOMIC BLOCK

All other things being equal, local anaesthetics block small nerves before large ones, so the sympathetic outflow (T1-L2) is particularly affected by spinal or epidural anaesthesia. Sympathetic blockade reduces vasomotor tone, causing vasodilatation. This in turn results in pooling of the blood, particularly in the legs, with a consequent decrease in venous return, cardiac output and blood pressure. The effect is analogous to the postural hypotension due to vasodilatation that occurs when stepping out of a hot bath. This fall in blood pressure is the most obvious unwanted effect of spinal and epidural anaesthesia; it is therefore mandatory to have intravenous access before performing the block and to have a vasoconstrictor drug such as ephedrine immediately available. It is also common practice to pre-load the circulation with 500–1000 mL of intravenous fluid.

SENSORY BLOCK

Essentially, sensory loss spreads outward from the dermatomes supplied by the spinal nerve closest to where the local anaesthetic is administered. Extent of spread, direction of spread (cranial or caudal) and laterality (left or right) can be influenced by the volume of local anaesthetic and posture of the patient, as will be seen later.

MOTOR BLOCK

Efferent motor fibres tend to be larger than sensory nerves, and so are blocked less effectively. However, spinal, and to a lesser extent epidural, anaesthesia causes profound motor weakness in the lower limbs. When anaesthesia needs to be extended high up the abdomen, as for Caesarean section, the motor block can affect the intercostal nerves, responsible for part of the work of breathing. Fortunately, the diaphragm, innervated by the phrenic nerve arising from C3-5, escapes all but the most dangerously high blocks and is quite able to maintain respiratory function. The arms, receiving their innervation from C5-T2, are also relatively immune to motor block.

Contraindications

Two potential hazards of inserting needles close to the central nervous system are haemorrhage causing cord compression, and infection. These blocks are not used, therefore, when a patient has clotting abnormalities (whether due to disease or drug therapy), or when there is septicaemia or local infection at the site of injection. Along with refusal by the patient and a history of sensitivity to local anaesthetics, these are the only absolute contraindications to spinal or epidural anaesthesia. However, the decreases in venous return and blood pressure already described mean that these techniques should be avoided in the shocked patient. Patients with myocardial ischaemia may also present a problem since, although vasodilatation means that the heart is pumping against less resistance, thus reducing cardiac work, the fall in diastolic blood pressure may reduce coronary artery perfusion.

Table 2.4 Spinal and epidural anaesthesia compared

Spinal anaesthesia	Epidural anaesthesia
Usually single injection through fine needle	Usually catheter passed through wide-bore needle —blunt needle → resistance
Small dose (1–3 mL)	Large dose (up to 20 mL)
Rapid onset	Slow onset
Dense, even block	May be patchy or even missing in some areas
Single shot means 'all or nothing'	Allows for further 'top-ups' to improve poor block
Duration of action limited by single dose	'Top-ups' allow for much longer duration
Risk of spinal headache	Headache only if accidental dural puncture
Rapid onset hypotension	Slow onset hypotension—easier to manage
Good for surgical procedures	Good for prolonged analgesia—labour/post-op

This section goes on to discuss some specific aspects of spinal and epidural blockade. A comparison of the two techniques is shown in Table 2.4.

Spinal Anaesthesia

Uses

Spinal anaesthesia produces a dense block of rapid onset with a duration dependent upon the drug used, two hours of useful operating time probably being the upper limit. It is particularly useful for surgical procedures below the waist, including hernia repair, prostatectomy and orthopaedic operations on the leg. Procedures involving extensive manipulation of abdominal organs are not normally suitable for spinal blockade, as the diffuse innervation of the peritoneum makes it difficult to block; there are many advantages, however, in avoiding general anaesthesia in obstetrics, and a sensory block up to T4 (the nipple line) allows Caesarean section to be performed with the mother (and father) actively participating in the birth. Blocks above this level are not really practical (Figure 2.4).

Spread of Block

As stated earlier, dural puncture is normally performed below L2 to minimize the risk of damaging the spinal cord. Since it is administered directly into the CSF, however, a small dose of local anaesthetic goes a long way – volumes exceeding 3 mL are rarely used. Spread of the drug within

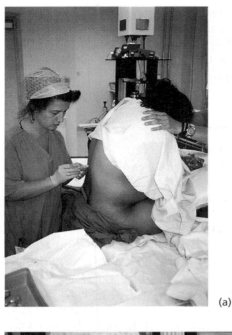

(a)

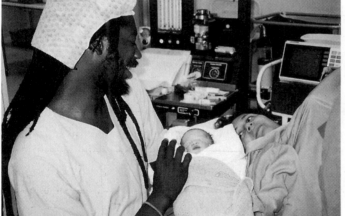

(b)

Figure 2.4 (a) Preparation of a patient for Caesarean section under spinal anaesthesia. (b) The happy family during the operation.

the CSF is determined largely by two interrelated factors – the baricity of the solution, and the posture of the patient.

Bupivacaine (0.5 per cent) is commonly used for spinal anaesthesia, and in its standard form is slightly hypobaric with respect to CSF. This means that, if CSF and bupivacaine were to be mixed in a tube, the drug would tend to float to the top. This property can be used to direct the spread of bupivacaine by positioning the patient after injection. Thus, putting the patient on his right side with head-up tilt will encourage blockade of the lower thoracic segments on the left – ideal for left inguinal hernia repair. 'Heavy' bupivacaine, dissolved in 8 per cent glucose, is also available; being markedly hyperbaric with respect to CSF, it acts in an opposite way to the plain solution. The use of heavy bupivacaine with the patient sitting up, for example, produces an excellent sacral block.

Spinal Headache

Although it permits injection of local anaesthetic, a hole in the dura mater also results in leakage of CSF into the epidural space after the needle has been withdrawn. This lowers the pressure of the CSF bathing the spinal cord and may cause a 'spinal' headache. Sometimes totally debilitating, spinal headache is exacerbated by any movement from the prone position or by bright lights, and may last for several weeks.

The incidence of headache is directly related to the size of the dural hole, and so very fine needles are normally used for spinal anaesthesia. Headache is also more common in young, female patients, and so is a particular problem following Caesarean section, when up to 10 per cent of patients may be affected. Treatment consists of lying flat in a darkened room, taking simple analgesics and encouraging fluid intake. If this is ineffective, a 'blood patch' may be performed, in which 20 mL of the patient's blood is injected into the epidural space, sealing the hole and producing instant relief. Modern needle technology has markedly reduced the incidence of headache, but it still remains the most common post-operative problem related to spinal anaesthesia.

Epidural Anaesthesia

Uses

Since the dura is not punctured during an epidural block, the need to use a fine needle to prevent spinal headache does not arise. The use of a wide-bore needle allows for the passage of a catheter into the epidural space, through which further doses of local anaesthetic can be given to prolong the duration of block. This is in marked contrast to the 'single-shot' spinal anaes-thetic with its strictly limited duration of action.

The presence of a catheter also means that a block can be 'built up' incre-mentally, monitoring the level of sensory loss throughout. A high block can be established relatively safely with better cardiovascular stability than with the sudden vasodilatation associated with a spinal technique.

What are the disadvantages of an epidural? The epidural space is filled with loose areolar tissue and blood vessels, and local anaesthetic does not spread as readily as when mixing with CSF in a spinal block. Due to this action, a single dose takes longer to work (20–30 minutes), the block may not be as dense as with a spinal, even leaving some dermatomes poorly anaesthetized, and a much larger dose of drug is needed (about 10 times the volume used for the equivalent spinal block). Epidural anaesthesia is suitable for any of the procedures for which spinal block is used, but the latter is usually preferred for its faster onset. Epidurals come into their own when a prolonged block is needed, in particular to relieve pain during labour, and are also being increasingly used to provide long-term post-operative analgesia. Since the site of insertion does not have to be confined to the lumbar region, thoracic epidurals can be used to provide analgesia following upper abdominal or chest surgery, and chronic neck problems can be relieved with a cervical epidural. The epidural space is also accessible in the caudal region, via the sacral hiatus; this route is particularly effective for perineal procedures such as penile circumcision.

Spread of the Block

In contrast to spinal block, posture has little effect on the spread of an epidural, and the baricity of the local anaesthetic solution is irrelevant. Volume of solution is all-important, and 20 mL or more may be needed to produce a block suitable for Caesarean section, bupivacaine usually being the drug of choice. Due to the ability to give further doses through the catheter, an incremental technique can be used to ensure an adequate block prior to surgery.

Inadvertent Dural Puncture

Location of the epidural space is not easy, and in 0.5–2 per cent of cases, the needle is accidentally advanced through the dura, a mishap signalled by a gush of CSF from the wide-bore needle. Dural puncture with such a large needle means that the chance of spinal headache is very high, and blood patch (see above) may well be needed.

If the dural puncture goes unrecognized, the anaesthetist may then administer a full epidural dose of local anaesthetic directly into the CSF. This results in a disastrous 'total spinal', where massive motor and sympathetic blockade usually lead to respiratory arrest, requiring immediate intervention.

Inadvertent Venous Catheterization

The catheter may be accidentally passed into one of the veins found in the epidural space – a particular risk in labour, as the epidural veins are dilated in the latter half of pregnancy. Administration of a full epidural dose of local anaesthetic in these circumstances results in toxic blood levels, with adverse effects on the central nervous and cardiovascular systems.

To reduce the risk of inadvertent subarachnoid or intravenous administration, the epidural catheter is aspirated before each dose to check for CSF or blood, and the dose of local anaesthetic is usually only given after a smaller 'test dose' has been administered.

Spinal and Epidural Opioids

Increasingly, opioids such as morphine, diamorphine and fentanyl are being given epidurally and spinally for post-operative analgesia. The idea is that, by directing these drugs to the receptor sites found in the substantia gelatinosa of the spinal cord, good-quality analgesia can be obtained with a smaller dose. These techniques have proved very effective following major abdominal and thoracic surgery. Concern about sudden, delayed-onset respiratory depression means that, in most centres, these techniques are only used in special high-dependency or intensive care areas.

Combined Regional and General Anaesthesia

Nerve blocks and epidurals are often used in conjunction with light general anaesthesia for operations where regional anaesthesia alone would be unsuitable. Such a combined approach means that lower doses of general anaesthetic agents may be used, and that good-quality afferent blockade is provided, minimizing the sympathetic responses to intra-operative pain. These patients enjoy improved cardiovascular stability during the procedure, recover and mobilize faster, and have less post-operative pain. When used with post-operative epidural opioids, the benefits of this technique can be tremendous.

Key Points

- Local/regional anaesthesia is gaining in popularity and is the technique of choice for many procedures.
- Toxicity of local anaesthetic solutions should always be borne in mind, and the maximum safe dose should be known whenever such drugs are used.
- The lowest suitable concentration should always be used.
- Patients should be fasted before major conduction blockade.
- Spinal anaesthesia produces a dense block with a rapid onset.
- Epidural analgesia has a slower onset time, but the potential for prolonging the block makes it more suitable for long procedures or in cases where post-operative analgesia is needed.

Further Reading

Brown, D.L. 1992: *Atlas of regional anesthesia*. Philadelphia: WB Saunders.
Cousins, M.J., Bridenbaugh, P.L. 1988: *Neural blockade in clinical anesthesia and management of pain* (2nd edn). Philadelphia: Lippincott.

3 Drugs Used in Anaesthesia

General Principles

Anaesthetists administer potent drugs of rapid onset, often with narrow safety margins. They give up to a dozen drugs in quick succession via a variety of routes, so it is not surprising that anaesthetists are expected to have a thorough knowledge of pharmacology. This comprises both pharmacokinetics ('what the body does to the drug') and pharmacodynamics ('what the drug does to the body').

Pharmacokinetics

Routes of Administration

Classically, anaesthetic drugs were administered by the inhalational route and, more recently, the intravenous route has been used for both induction and maintenance. Nowadays, virtually any route may be used and examples are given in Table 3.1.

Drug Distribution

Most anaesthetic drugs are necessarily lipid soluble since they are required to act in the central nervous system and therefore have to cross the blood–brain barrier, a barrier composed mostly of lipid membrane. The important exception to this rule is the group of muscle relaxant drugs, which are water soluble since they do not act in the central nervous system.

Drug Elimination

Elimination of drugs occurs classically by metabolism or renal excretion, although in the case of the inhalational anaesthetic agents excretion of unchanged drug occurs through the lungs.

Table 3.1 Routes of administration of anaesthetic drugs

Route	Examples
Intravenous	Induction agents, muscle relaxants, opioid analgesics
Inhalational	Volatile anaesthetics, nitrous oxide
Intramuscular	Opioids for post-operative analgesia
Subcutaneous	Opioids for post-operative analgesia
Intrathecal/epidural	Local anaesthetics, opioids
Rectal	Diclofenac
Topical to skin	EMLA[a]
Transdermal	Hyoscine
Sublingual	Buprenorphine
Nasal	Sufentanil
Nerve plexus/local infiltration	Local anaesthetics

[a]Eutectic mixture of local anaesthetics.

Simple chemistry suggests that water-soluble drugs are eliminated by renal excretion, and this applies to most muscle relaxants. The important exceptions are the depolarizing agent suxamethonium (which is metabolized by plasma cholinesterase in the blood) and the non-depolarizing agent atracurium (which breaks down spontaneously at blood pH and temperature).

Most other anaesthetic drugs, such as the intravenous induction agents and the opioid analgesics, are lipid soluble and so undergo hepatic metabolism. It is important to appreciate, however, that the duration of action of many intravenous induction agents does not depend on the rate of metabolism and this applies particularly to thiopentone. Thiopentone is metabolized slowly, and its short duration of action depends instead on the phenomenon of redistribution; the initial bolus of drug is distributed preferentially to the brain because of the distribution of cardiac output, then almost immediately begins to diffuse out of the brain as it is redistributed to other tissues (such as muscle) which receive less of the cardiac output.

Inhalational agents, while primarily excreted through the lungs, undergo a variable degree of hepatic metabolism and this may have clinical consequences (see below).

Volumes of Distribution, Compartments and Elimination Half-lives

These considerations are important in deciding the dose of a drug for an individual patient, the frequency of administration and the likely duration of action – a particularly important point for the anaesthetist, whose drugs are required to terminate their action at a fixed time.

Pharmacodynamics

Drugs may act by a variety of mechanisms. Important among these are:

1. Drugs which act by virtue of their physico-chemical properties. The classic examples of these are desferrioxamine and calcium resonium, which act by chelation of iron and potassium, respectively. Examples in anaesthetic practice are less clear. Local anaesthetic agents are believed to act by altering the internal aspect of the sodium channel in the neuronal cell membrane. Inhalational anaesthetics depend partly for their action on lipid solubility, the more potent agents being more lipid soluble; however, this relationship is not invariable and does not account for all their properties.
2. Drugs which act by inhibition of enzyme systems. A classic example in anaesthetic practice is the use of anticholinesterases to reverse the effect of neuromuscular blocking drugs (see below).
3. Drugs which act by interaction with specific receptors. There are several examples in anaesthetic practice, including competitive neuromuscular blocking drugs, opioid analgesics and antimuscarinic drugs such as atropine. Often these act by classic competitive antagonism (i.e. the effect may be reversed by excess of agonist) and this explains why some aspects of a general anaesthetic (neuromuscular blockade, narcotic analgesia) may be 'reversed' while others (unconsciousness, local anaesthesia) cannot.

Drug Interactions in Anaesthesia

These are discussed in Chapter 6.

Individual Drugs

The following is not intended to be an exhaustive account of the properties of each agent, but an attempt to highlight those properties which affect the way the drug is used.

Drugs Used for Premedication

The subject of premedication is discussed in more detail in Chapter 6. Benzodiazepines remain the most popular choice, and it makes sense to use one with a relatively short half-life, such as temazepam. They are usually given orally for convenience and comfort.

Intravenous Induction Agents

These may be defined as drugs which produce reversible unconsciousness, commonly in one arm–brain circulation time. Their duration of action is usually short and they are most commonly used as a rapid, pleasant way of starting anaesthesia before continuing with an inhalational agent.

THIOPENTONE

Thiopentone, a short-acting barbiturate, has been in use for more than fifty years and remains the standard against which other agents are compared. The properties of the barbiturate ring and the structure–activity relationships of the barbiturates represent a fascinating example of applied pharmacology, and the interested reader is referred to more detailed books on general pharmacology.

In common with other barbiturates, thiopentone causes respiratory and cardiovascular depression – in other words, the patient may stop breathing and the blood pressure may fall, sometimes dramatically. These are rarely a major problem in the patient who is otherwise fit, but may be significant (and potentially fatal) in, for example, the patient who is hypovolaemic, elderly or has severe heart disease.

METHOHEXITONE

This is another short-acting barbiturate with many properties similar to thiopentone. Unlike thiopentone, it has convulsant properties and so is contraindicated in epileptic patients.

ETOMIDATE

This is a non-barbiturate induction agent whose most desirable property is stability of the cardiovascular system. Many anaesthetists regard it as the agent of choice in the hypovolaemic patient, the patient with severe cardiac disease and sometimes the elderly patient. Injection tends to be painful.

PROPOFOL

This is another non-barbiturate induction agent, characterized by rapid recovery and non-cumulation. Unlike thiopentone, it can therefore be given in repeated doses or by infusion over prolonged periods. It is often used for day-case surgery (where rapid recovery is obviously desirable) and by infusion in situations where administration of a volatile anaesthetic is impossible or undesirable (for example, during bronchoscopy or in patients with susceptibility to malignant hyperpyrexia). It has also found a place when given by continuous infusion for sedation in intensive care. Propofol obtunds laryngeal and pharyngeal reflexes better than do other agents, so is often used for induction when a laryngeal mask airway (see Chapter 1) is to be inserted during spontaneous breathing. Respiratory and cardiovascular depression occur.

KETAMINE

This has various unique characteristics compared with other induction agents. There is little cardiovascular or respiratory depression and muscle tone is retained. It is an effective analgesic in relatively small doses, and is a potent bronchodilator.

The main disadvantage of ketamine is the occurrence of emergence phenomena, characteristically unpleasant nightmares. Although the incidence and severity of these may be reduced by allowing the patient to recover in a quiet environment, they are troublesome enough to preclude the use of ketamine in all except very compelling circumstances. On balance, ketamine is rarely indicated in modern anaesthesia but when it is indicated there is no substitute and there are few anaesthetists who have not been grateful for the existence of ketamine at least once during their career! It is used quite extensively in third world countries because it is cheap, convenient to use, and obviates the need for complex apparatus.

Muscle Relaxants

Muscle relaxants are divided into two groups: competitive (or non-depolarizing) and non-competitive (or depolarizing). These terms give a clear idea of the mode of action of these drugs. Competitive relaxants work by straightforward competitive antagonism of acetylcholine at the neuromuscular junction, while non-competitive relaxants work by causing prolonged depolarization of the muscle membrane so that nerve impulses and acetylcholine release are unable to initiate muscle contraction. The use of anticholinesterases is intimately associated with the use of muscle relaxants, so these drugs are also discussed here.

COMPETITIVE MUSCLE RELAXANTS

The original example of this group of drugs was curare which, as every schoolboy knows, was originally discovered being used as a South American arrow poison. Less well known is the fact that, as long ago as the early nineteenth century, it was demonstrated that animals poisoned with curare could be kept alive by artificial ventilation; it took more than a hundred years for this simple observation to be applied in anaesthesia and intensive care, a salutary lesson for those tempted to dismiss results which seem to have no immediate relevance. Curare itself is still occasionally used in clinical practice, and is still imported from the headwaters of the Amazon (there being no manufacturing process), but it has been almost entirely superseded by newer competitive muscle relaxants.

The main problems with curare are its cardiovascular side-effects (hypotension) and its relatively long duration of action (approximately 40 minutes). The aim of the development of the competitive muscle relaxants has been to try to eliminate side-effects and reduce the duration of action. A list of most of the competitive muscle relaxants in current use is given in Table 3.2, together with the duration of action and other properties. The duration of action is usually taken to be the time interval between giving a dose large enough to permit tracheal intubation and being able to reverse the residual blockade (see below).

Table 3.2 Competitive muscle relaxants in common use

Drug	Duration of action (min)	Other properties
d-Tubocurarine	40	Causes hypotension by histamine release and ganglion blockade
Pancuronium	45	May cause tachycardia and hypertension
Vecuronium	15–20	Few side-effects
Atracurium	15–20	Elimination is independent of renal and hepatic function
M vacurium	10–15	Recently introduced
Rocuronium	15–20	Recently introduced
Cisatracurium	40	Recently introduced

The choice of muscle relaxant for a particular procedure is made by considering the required duration of action, side-effect profile and the effect of any co-existing disease (for example, atracurium is often chosen in patients with renal failure since its elimination is independent of renal function). The current trend is to prefer the shorter-acting relaxants such as atracurium and vecuronium, and give repeated increments or an infusion for longer procedures. Doses may be titrated accurately by monitoring neuromuscular function with a peripheral nerve stimulator (see Chapter 5).

ANTICHOLINESTERASES

At the end of surgery, it would be possible simply to continue ventilating the lungs artificially until the muscle relaxant has completely worn off. This would, however, be hazardous for the patient and would present an impossible load to the recovery ward, so this is only done in the rare instances when artificial ventilation is to be continued on an intensive care unit. For all other patients, we make use of the important property of competitive relaxants: the effects may be overcome by excess of agonist. The agonist in this case is, of course, acetylcholine. It is dangerous and impractical to give acetylcholine itself so instead we inhibit the breakdown of acetylcholine by giving an anticholinesterase. Neostigmine is the one used most commonly as it has a convenient duration of action and does not cross the blood–brain barrier; edrophonium, another anticholinesterase drug, is used occasionally. The other anticholinesterases, physostigmine and pyridostigmine, have little application in anaesthesia.

By inhibiting the breakdown of acetylcholine, the effects of this transmitter will be increased wherever acetylcholine is found, at least outside the central nervous system. Most importantly, transmission from post-ganglionic parasympathetic fibres to the effector organ is exaggerated and this produces a number of side-effects. Most significant among these is bradycardia, which may proceed to sinus arrest. It is obviously essential to counteract these side-effects, and this is where the sustained efforts of physiologists to categorize acetylcholine receptors bears obvious fruit. We want to maintain the action of acetylcholine at the nicotinic receptors (the neuromuscular junction) but impair its actions at muscarinic receptors (the parasympathetic effector organ junction, particularly the vagus nerve and the heart). So, we give an anti-muscarinic drug such as atropine whenever an anticholinesterase is administered. Atropine was used for this purpose for many years, but recently, glycopyrrolate has been preferred, mainly because its duration of action is closer to that of neostigmine.

This explains the logic of giving a mixture of neostigmine and glycopyrrolate at the end of surgery. Residual paralysis is reversed, and muscle power restored sufficiently for the patient to breathe and cough effectively.

NON-COMPETITIVE MUSCLE RELAXANTS

As mentioned above, these relaxants work by inducing prolonged depolarization of the muscle membrane. This produces an initial contraction of muscle, manifested clinically as the unco-ordinated contractions known as fasciculations, which last a few seconds before profound paralysis occurs. Paralysis then normally lasts up to about five minutes.

The only non-competitive muscle relaxant in clinical use at present is suxamethonium. Its onset of action is faster than that of any competitive relaxant, so it is used when it is necessary to pass a tracheal tube as soon as possible after induction of anaesthesia – typically, in a rapid-sequence induction when the patient is at risk of regurgitation of stomach contents (see Chapter 1). The other main indication for suxamethonium is when the trachea is to be intubated and then the patient allowed to breathe spontaneously – as, for example, during ENT surgery.

While suxamethonium usually lasts about 5 minutes, there is a small group of patients in the population who metabolize the drug excessively slowly because of abnormal plasma cholinesterase (the enzyme responsible for the breakdown of suxamethonium) in their blood. In these patients, the duration of action may be up to 24 hours (although it is usually 20–240 minutes). This state is sometimes termed 'scoline apnoea' (scoline being one of the trade names for suxamethonium). This is not a major problem provided that the situation is appreciated and arrangements made for prolonged mechanical ventilation and sedation, either in a recovery ward or an intensive care unit. The patient and family will require information and advice.

The main disadvantages of suxamethonium are the incidence of severe muscle pains post-operatively (which tend to be particularly bad in the ambulant patient), and the occurrence of bradycardia, especially in the neonate and after repeated doses in the adult.

Analgesics

Analgesic, or pain-killing, drugs are divided into two main groups, opioid analgesics and anti-inflammatory analgesics. Generally, opioids are used for more severe pain such as that which follows major surgery, while anti-inflammatory agents are used for less severe pain. Local anaesthetics are also used for their pain-killing properties but are discussed separately below. Other aspects of analgesia are discussed in Chapter 7.

OPIOID ANALGESICS

Terminology needs to be clarified. *Opiates* are the naturally occurring alkaloids of the opium poppy. *Opioids* are all drugs, occurring naturally or manufactured, which have the properties of this class of drug. The term 'opioid' is therefore more general. The properties of opioids are given in Table 3.3. Opioid pharmacology has been given impetus by the discovery of opioid receptors in the CNS and the isolation of endogenous ligands (substances such as endorphins which bind to the receptors). Receptor sub-types have been identified, and it is hoped that further work will allow the separation of the 'desirable' properties of opioids (particularly analgesia) from the 'undesirable' ones such as respiratory depression and nausea and vomiting. It is likely to be some time before this 'Holy Grail' is attained, if it is achievable at all.

The classic and original example of this group of drugs is morphine, which has been used medicinally for hundreds of years. Other compounds, such as diamorphine and pethidine, have been produced in attempts to reduce the side-effects but none of these drugs has been demonstrated to have signifi-cant advantages over morphine. The major use of these drugs is, of course, for analgesia. For this purpose they may be given by virtually any route imaginable: intravenous, intramuscular, subcutaneous, epidural or intrathe-cal for acute post-operative pain, and oral, sublingual or rectal for chronic cancer pain. Post-operative pain is discussed in detail in Chapter 7. Their other common use is for analgesia and sedation in ventilated patients on the intensive care unit.

Morphine is an example of a *pure agonist* opioid. As the term suggests, this means that it activates opioid receptors and has no antagonist properties. Most of the commonly used opioids are pure agonists.

Some opioids are *partial agonists*. Examples include buprenorphine and pentazocine. These drugs bind to opioid receptors but fail to elicit a complete response. There are few uses for partial agonists in anaesthesia.

Finally, there is a group of opioids which are classed as *pure antagonists*. The only example in clinical use is naloxone. This drug binds to opioid recep-tors without eliciting a response and thereby acts as a classic competitive

Table 3.3 Some properties of opioids

Analgesia—intracranial action
Analgesia—spinal action
Sedation
Respiratory depression
Nausea and vomiting
Miosis
Constipation
Urinary retention
Itching
Contraction of the Sphincter of Oddi

antagonist. Its clinical use is to reverse the side-effects of excessive opioid administration, either in the accident and emergency department (where the overdose may be self-inflicted) or in the ward (where the patient has proved more sensitive to the drug than was expected). There are two problems with naloxone. First, it takes a few minutes to achieve its full effect so that it is easy to give too much and thus reverse the (desired) analgesia as well as the (undesired) respiratory depression. It is easy to state 'the dose must be titrated carefully' but this is difficult to do when you are confronted with a hypoxic, apnoeic patient at 2 a.m.! The other problem is its relatively short duration of action, about 30 minutes. Most opioids have a duration of action considerably longer than this, and it is often necessary to give a further dose of naloxone, or to give it by infusion for a period of time.

ANTI-INFLAMMATORY ANALGESICS

Commonly known as non-steroidal anti-inflammatory drugs or NSAIDs, these are usually described as having three properties: anti-inflammatory, analgesic and antipyretic. Each individual drug possesses these properties in differing degrees, and the ones most commonly used in anaesthesia possess primarily analgesic properties. Their mode of action is by inhibition of prostaglandin synthesis in the tissues – a peripheral action, in contrast to the central action of the opioids.

NSAIDs may be used as analgesics in their own right after minor surgery. After major surgery they are increasingly being used for the 'opioid-sparing' action. This means that, by giving one of these agents, less opioid is required to achieve a given degree of analgesia, with a consequent reduction in the severity of side-effects. Naturally there is a price to pay for this convenience, and NSAIDs have their own side-effects, including bronchospasm, renal impairment and clotting abnormalities; thus there is a significant number of patients in whom their use is contraindicated.

Examples of NSAIDs in common use in anaesthesia include diclofenac (which is most conveniently given orally or by suppository) and ketorolac (which may be given orally, intramuscularly or intravenously).

Inhalational Anaesthetics

The original anaesthetic was an inhaled agent and for nearly a hundred years the inhalational agents ether, chloroform and nitrous oxide were the only anaesthetics in common use. Ether and chloroform have now been abandoned, ether because of its flammability and chloroform because of unacceptable side-effects, but nitrous oxide retains an important place in anaesthetic practice. Other potent inhalational agents are used nowadays to maintain anaesthesia, usually following intravenous induction.

GENERAL PRINCIPLES

While induction of anaesthesia takes place almost invariably (except in young children) by the intravenous route and is maintained by the inhalational

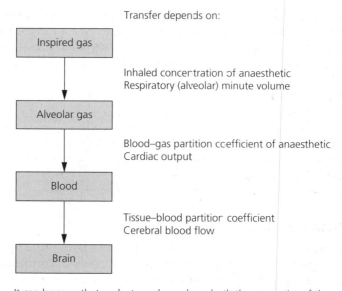

Transfer depends on:

Inspired gas

Inhaled concentration of anaesthetic
Respiratory (alveolar) minute volume

Alveolar gas

Blood–gas partition coefficient of anaesthetic
Cardiac output

Blood

Tissue–blood partition coefficient
Cerebral blood flow

Brain

It can be seen that each stage depends on both the properties of the anaesthetic agent and the physiological state of the patient.

Figure 3.1 Stages in the transfer of inhalational anaesthetic agents from inhaled gas mixture to the brain.

route, it is still important that the inhalational agent should achieve an adequate depth of anaesthesia quickly. This is partly for convenience, but there are also important clinical reasons. The patient does not wish to recover consciousness after the effects of the induction agent have worn off and before adequate anaesthesia is achieved with the inhalational agent. In addition, the depth of anaesthesia should be rapidly controllable during anaesthesia to take account of changing circumstances (such as haemorrhage or the intensity of surgical stimulus).

In order to achieve anaesthesia, the agent must be present in the brain in sufficient concentration. It must therefore pass from inspired gas to alveolar gas, from alveolar gas to blood and from blood to brain. Each of these steps requires different chemical properties (solubility in different tissues) so that the overall picture is complex. Figure 3.1 represents the process, which may be summarized as: agents of high solubility (in blood) give a slow induction, the speed of which depends mainly on ventilation, while agents of low solubility give a rapid induction, the speed of which is influenced mainly by cardiac output.

It is usual clinical practice to attain a given depth of anaesthesia as rapidly as possible and then to maintain the same depth for the rest of the operation. This is done by giving a relatively high inspired concentration of agent to begin with, followed by a decreasing concentration until equilibrium is achieved – complete equilibrium would take some hours but in practice the *inspired* concentration is reduced over the first ten or fifteen minutes and then kept constant, to produce a rapid increase in brain concentration, followed by a relatively steady concentration.

Elimination of inhaled anaesthetic agents is a 'mirror image' of uptake. Recovery, therefore, is more rapid with the less soluble agents.

INDIVIDUAL AGENTS

When discussing individual inhalational agents it is important to have a clear idea of relative potency. Potency is normally expressed as minimum alveolar concentration or MAC: this is defined as the minimum alveolar concentration which prevents reflex movement in response to skin incision in 50 per cent of subjects. It is important to appreciate that the MAC value does not tell you the 'right' concentration of agent to give. Firstly, the MAC value is affected by many variables such as age and the presence of other drugs such as premedicants or analgesics, and secondly, the anaesthetist's reputation tends to suffer if half his patients move when the surgeon starts his operation! The main value of the MAC concept is to compare the potencies of different agents.

The potency of anaesthetic agents is related to their lipid solubility (often expressed as the oil/gas partition coefficient). The greater the lipid solubility, the greater the potency and the lower the MAC value. Table 3.4 gives these variables for the commonly used inhalational agents, together with their blood/gas partition coefficients ('solubility') which, as discussed above, determine the speed of induction and recovery. The properties and uses of the individual agents will be discussed in the light of this information.

All the potent anaesthetic vapours share certain properties, mainly depression of the cardiovascular system (causing hypotension) and respiratory depression, although they possess these properties in differing degrees. These agents also lack any useful analgesic properties.

Table 3.4 Some properties of individual inhalational agents

| | Partition coefficients | | Oil/gas | MAC (%)[a] | % Met[b] |
	Blood/gas	Brain/blood			
Halothane	2.3	6.5	220	0.75	20
Enflurane	1.7	1.4	98	1.7	2
Isoflurane	1.4	2.5	98	1.2	0.2
Nitrous oxide	0.47	1.2	1.4	105	—
Sevoflurane	0.69		47	1.7	5
Desflurane	0.42		20	6.0	0.02

[a]MAC values are those in 100% oxygen.
[b]Met is the percentage of the inhaled vapour which undergoes hepatic metabolism.
Note that as the lipid solubility (oil/gas partition coefficient) falls, so does the potency (MAC rises).

NITROUS OXIDE

With a MAC value of over 100 per cent (this figure is obtained by extrapolation), it is clearly impossible to achieve satisfactory anaesthesia with nitrous oxide alone. It remains useful in conjunction with the more potent anaesthetic vapours since its presence reduces the MAC value of these agents. A lower alveolar concentration of these agents is often safer, because all of them depress the cardiovascular and respiratory systems to a much greater degree than does nitrous oxide.

Nitrous oxide must be used in high concentrations (50–70 per cent) to have any value. Being present in such high concentrations, it has unique side-effects. For example, although less soluble in blood than most other anaesthetic agents, it is more soluble than nitrogen, and this has two major consequences. First, nitrous oxide diffuses into air-filled body cavities faster than nitrogen diffuses out so that it causes expansion of compliant spaces such as the gut and an increased pressure in less compliant spaces such as the pleural cavity (in the presence of a pneumothorax). Second, when nitrous oxide is discontinued at the end of anaesthesia, it diffuses into the alveoli faster than nitrogen diffuses from alveoli into blood, and the resulting dilution of alveolar oxygen is termed 'diffusion hypoxia'; this may contribute to post-operative hypoxia for the first 5–10 minutes after the end of the anaesthetic.

Although it is unsuitable alone for use as an *anaesthetic*, nitrous oxide does have useful *analgesic* properties. It is available as a 50 per cent mixture with oxygen as 'Entonox' and is extensively used in midwifery, at accident sites and during post-operative chest physiotherapy.

HALOTHANE

Halothane has some potentially useful properties. It is the least irritant of the potent anaesthetic vapours, which makes it appropriate for use in inhalational induction, both in small children and in the occasional adult who requires an inhalational induction. It is a potent bronchodilator, which may make it the agent of choice in asthmatic patients.

A significant disadvantage is that it sensitizes the myocardium to the effects of catecholamines. Put more plainly, it makes it more likely that arrhythmias will develop during states of high circulating catecholamine levels – for example, when the surgeon has infiltrated the surgical site with adrenaline to produce a bloodless field, or when severe respiratory depression occurs.

Virtually every medical student has heard of 'halothane hepatitis', which is a severe inflammatory reaction of the liver in response to exposure to halothane. It is very rare (occurring perhaps once in every 20 000–50 000 halothane anaesthetics), most commonly follows repeat exposure to halothane, and may be fatal. Its existence has led to the recommendation that halothane should be avoided within 3 months of a previous halothane anaesthetic (since this is the period of greatest risk) and has also contributed to its decline in popularity in recent years.

ENFLURANE

This has proved to be a useful all-purpose inhalational anaesthetic. Perhaps the one property which distinguishes it is its tendency to produce epileptiform appearances on the EEG, and it is therefore usually avoided in epileptic patients.

ISOFLURANE

This agent reduces cardiac output less than the other two potent agents and it is often preferred in patients with cardiac failure. Isoflurane also produces more arteriolar vasodilatation than the other two agents, so it has found a use in operations requiring induced hypotension. Its physical properties, particularly its low solubility in blood, predict that it would have a rapid onset and offset of action. However, the irritant nature of the vapour means that, with a spontaneously breathing patient, the inspired concentration can be increased only slowly compared with halothane or enflurane, so it has not proved quite as useful in day-case anaesthesia as was hoped.

DESFLURANE

Introduced relatively recently into clinical practice in the UK, its properties suggest that it may be particularly useful when rapid onset or recovery is required. A drawback is its low boiling point, which means that it must be delivered from a special sort of vaporizer with a power supply which keeps the agent at a constant temperature in the vapour phase. Another disadvantage is that it is irritant to the respiratory tract, making it unsuitable for gas induction.

SEVOFLURANE

This is another new volatile anaesthetic agent in the UK, although it has been in use for some years in Japan. Like desflurane, sevoflurane has a low blood/gas solubility coefficient, resulting in rapid onset and rapid recovery. However, unlike desflurane, it is neither pungent nor irritant to the respiratory tract, and is therefore an extremely useful agent for gas induction, e.g. in children or in patients with difficult veins. In addition, it can be delivered from a conventional vaporizer. Sevoflurane is likely to become popular, particularly in paediatric anaesthesia.

METABOLISM OF INHALATIONAL AGENTS

Clearly, the main route of elimination of the inhalational agents is via the lungs. However, all of the potent agents discussed above undergo a degree of hepatic metabolism or 'biotransformation'. In the case of halothane this may be considerable (Table 3.4) and the metabolites are believed to play a role in the pathogenesis of 'halothane hepatitis'. Methoxyflurane is a volatile agent which is no longer used because the free fluoride ions generated by metabolism cause renal failure. It is obvious from Table 3.4 that desflurane has the lowest rate of biotransformation so is least likely to generate toxic metabolites.

Local Anaesthetic Agents

A local anaesthetic may be defined as a drug which reversibly blocks nerve conduction when applied locally in an appropriate concentration. Agents such as phenol and alcohol are therefore excluded from this definition since their action is irreversible.

LOCAL EFFECTS

There is reversible blockade of nerve conduction by the action termed 'membrane stabilization', the duration of which depends on the individual agent. There is also a local effect on the blood vessels; cocaine causes vasoconstriction while procaine causes vasodilatation and the rest have a minor vasodilator effect. Vasoconstrictors such as adrenaline may be added to the latter groups to reduce systemic absorption and thereby increase the duration of action and reduce the risk of systemic toxicity. Vasoconstrictors are not added to cocaine.

REGIONAL EFFECTS

Blockade of sympathetic fibres produces vasodilatation. This may be desirable, for example, in arm surgery on blood vessels when an arterio-venous fistula is being created for haemodialysis. In other situations it is less desirable and may be harmful, causing, for example, the significant hypotension which may accompany spinal anaesthesia.

SYSTEMIC EFFECTS

(i) CNS effects

These occur when an excessive amount of drug enters the circulation, either because an excessive dose has been infiltrated locally or because an appropriate amount has been given but has erroneously been injected into a blood vessel instead of the tissues. There is a brief period of sedation (which may be absent if the build-up of local anaesthetic is rapid) which is followed by convulsions and sometimes by brainstem depression. Treatment is largely supportive, ensuring oxygenation and adequate ventilation, but anticonvulsants may be required and a period of intensive care may be necessary if brainstem effects are present.

(ii) Cardiac effects

There is a membrane stabilizing action on cardiac tissue, which accounts for the therapeutic use of lignocaine in the treatment of ventricular ectopic activity. There is also depression of myocardial contractility, which is particularly marked with bupivacaine.

The clinical uses of local anaesthetic agents are discussed in Chapter 2.

4 Anaesthetic Equipment

Introduction

Although the modern anaesthetist is often viewed by his medical colleagues as a slave to technology, unable to function without a panoply of expensive equipment, it was not always thus. The ultimate in simplicity was probably achieved by James Young Simpson, Professor of Midwifery at Edinburgh University, who in 1847 used chloroform dripped onto a piece of gauze held near the patient's face to relieve the pain of labour. This 'low-tech' approach rapidly gained favour, and was even used by John Snow to administer chloroform to Queen Victoria for the birth of Prince Leopold in 1853. 'Rag and bottle' anaesthesia, with minor modifications, remained popular well into the 20th century, and lives on today in low-budget Hollywood spy movies, where the hero is incapacitated by the bad guys clamping a chloroform-soaked handkerchief over his face – bad guys, of course, because they have frequently failed to observe the most basic precautions of pre-operative fasting before inducing anaesthesia.

There are some areas of anaesthetic practice where simplicity remains at a premium, and here the vestiges of low-technology anaesthesia can still be witnessed. In the armed forces, where surgery may have to be performed in the field, portability is the most vital property, and anaesthetic equipment such as the Triservice apparatus is standard issue. The luxury of compressed gas is often beyond the means of developing countries, and reliance is placed on simple 'drawover' vaporizers which add agents such as ether to inspired atmospheric air.

In general, though, modern anaesthesia needs a somewhat more sophisticated approach. The recognition that oxygen enrichment of the inspired gas mixture is needed to prevent hypoxia and the widespread adoption of nitrous oxide as an anaesthetic agent have resulted in the need for pressurized gas supplies wherever anaesthesia is administered, and this has shaped the development of apparatus. The introduction of powerful volatile agents has meant that accurate delivery systems are necessary to prevent overdosage. The complexity of modern surgery, allied to the widespread use of muscle relaxants, has forced the introduction of better methods of airway management. Finally, the recognition of the possible hazards of chronic exposure to low levels of anaesthetic agents has led to the development of methods for removing waste gases and vapours from the vicinity of the operating theatre.

Anaesthetic Gases

Modern general anaesthetic practice is totally dependent on a reliable supply of compressed oxygen and, to a lesser extent, nitrous oxide. The anaesthetist faced with a loss of compressed gas to a paralysed patient must very rapidly find an alternative method of ventilating the lungs. In these circumstances a self-inflating bag, of the type used for resuscitation, must be immediately to hand, and many anaesthetists have, on these rare occasions, resorted to the expedient of blowing down the tracheal tube in desperation while waiting for this simple piece of equipment. Other compressed gases, such as air and carbon dioxide, are often supplied in the modern operating theatre.

Pipelines

Nearly all anaesthetic machines are supplied with gas via pipelines which emerge from the wall or ceiling of the operating theatre (Figure 4.1). These originate elsewhere in the hospital either from a large bank of cylinders (in the case of nitrous oxide) or from a tank of liquid oxygen. The contents of a pipeline are easily identifiable from its labelling and colour-coding, but the implications of the pipelines carrying the wrong gas are so serious that strict precautions are taken to ensure that misconnection cannot occur anywhere from the gas supply right into the anaesthetic machine. A particular hazard is cross-connection, where the oxygen and nitrous oxide pipelines are accidentally swapped; when a mixture of the two gases is being used, there is little out of the ordinary to be seen, but the act of switching off the 'nitrous oxide' and increasing the flow of 'oxygen' at the end of an operation results in the onset of hypoxia which can prove fatal if the cause is not quickly identified.

Cylinders

The vital importance of a pressurized supply of oxygen is such that the pipeline is never relied upon, and at least one full cylinder of oxygen is always immediately available on the anaesthetic machine. A backup cylinder of nitrous oxide is also available, and the carbon dioxide supply (if fitted) is usually served by a cylinder. Other cylinders may include air or even cyclopropane (now rarely used). With all this potential for confusion, it is important that misconnection cannot occur, and this is ensured by an international system of colour-coding and the use of the 'pin-index' system which keys each cylinder to its respective yoke (Figure 4.1). Even then, mistakes can occur; in Hong Kong in the late 1980s a patient died during routine surgery – the cause of death was found to be an oxygen cylinder on the anaesthetic machine which contained pure nitrogen.

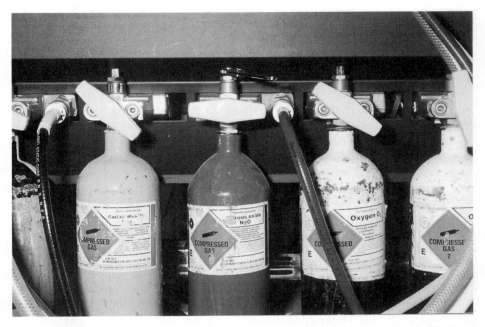

Figure 4.1 Pipeline and cylinder connections on the back of an anaesthetic machine.

The Anaesthetic Machine

Although the modern anaesthetic machine bears little resemblance to the apparatus first designed by Edmund Boyle in 1917, its functions are remarkably similar. In essence, the purpose of the anaesthetic machine is to provide a supply of compressed gas, to regulate the pressure of the gas, to allow mixing of the gases in varying proportions and flows, to enable controlled addition of a volatile agent, to deliver the final mixture to a common gas outlet, and to provide a surface on which the anaesthetist can lay his equipment, drugs and record.

Pressure and Flow

Anaesthetic machines are designed to function at a pressure of 400 kPa (or 4 atmospheres or 60 lb/in²; there are more units for measuring pressure than there are minutes in a surgeon's hour). Pipeline gas is supplied at this pressure and so can be delivered directly to the flowmeters. Cylinder pressure, however, is higher (5000 kPa for a full nitrous oxide cylinder and 12 000 kPa for oxygen) and tends to fall as the cylinder empties. Pressure regulators are therefore interposed between the cylinders and the flowmeters.

Each gas passes to a dedicated flowmeter (Figure 4.2), which allows the operator to control the flow of the gas into the backbar (the part of the machine in which the gases mix and upon which the vaporizer is mounted).

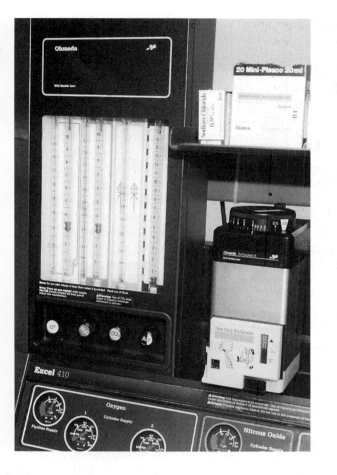

Figure 4.2 Fascia of a modern anaesthetic machine, showing flowmeter bank and enflurane vaporizer.

The set flow rate is indicated on most machines by a spinning bobbin in a glass tube; the rotation of the bobbin confirms that it is floating freely in the tube rather than stuck to the side. By tradition, in the UK the oxygen flow control knob is shaped differently from the others so that it can be identified in the event of a blackout and oxygen is always located on the far left of the bank of flowmeters. In fact, this position for the oxygen is not ideal, as any crack in the glass of the flowmeter bank will tend to preferentially spill oxygen, resulting in a hypoxic mixture. Modern machines get around this problem by channelling the oxygen flow into the backbar beyond its point of connection with the flowmeters (see below).

Vaporizers

Anaesthetic agents like halothane and isoflurane are liquids with low boiling points; passing gas over them picks up vapour from the surface of the liquid and adds the vapour to the gas mixture. The amount of vapour picked up is related to the nature of the interface between the gas and the liquid and the temperature within the vaporizing chamber. When ether and trichlorethylene were popular agents it was sufficient to put them in a simple glass bottle with an unsophisticated control for splitting the gas flow so that only part of it entered the bottle, but nowadays more care must be taken. At room temperature and pressure, halothane can reach a concentration of 33 per cent in a gas mixture. Halothane is effective at concentrations as low as 0.75 per cent, and has powerful respiratory and cardiovascular effects at higher levels, and so it is important that modern vaporizers are reliable and accurate.

One of the main problems with ensuring accurate delivery of a vapour is that, as vaporization occurs, the temperature of the liquid drops. This means that the concentration delivered by the vaporizer will tend to fall as time goes by. One method of compensating for this is apparent as soon as you pick up a modern vaporizer; its surprising weight is due to a thick coat of copper which acts as a 'heat sink', drawing heat into the vaporizer from the atmosphere. Further compensation is provided by a temperature-sensitive internal mechanism which alters the relative gas flows through the vapour chamber and bypass mechanism to allow for loss of heat. To prevent the inadvertent administration of more than one powerful volatile agent, most vaporizer systems incorporate a device which only allows one vaporizer to be turned on at a time. Add to this a keyed filling port to prevent atmospheric pollution or use of the wrong agent and a high-resistance internal pathway to prevent gas being 'blown-back' through the vaporizer by the pressure wave generated by a ventilator, and it is apparent that the modern vaporizer is a precision, high-technology piece of equipment. This is taken to extremes by the new vaporizer which has been developed for use with desflurane; the physical properties of this agent are such that the vaporizer has its own power supply to heat and pressurize the contents.

Modern Modifications

Safety requirements for anaesthetic machines have become more stringent during the last decade, and modern machines reflect these concerns by incorporating several modifications, such as the preferential oxygen delivery device mentioned above.

Oxygen failure alarms, which alert the anaesthetist to a drop in pressure in the oxygen supply, have been with us for a while, but a recent improvement has been hypoxic mixture prevention. As its name suggests, this device prevents delivery of a mixture containing less than 25–30 per cent oxygen by linking the oxygen and nitrous oxide control knobs.

All machines incorporate oxygen flush mechanisms for rapidly providing 100 per cent oxygen in an emergency, but these are not without their hazards. If the flush is inadvertently left open, the anaesthetic mixture is diluted and intraoperative awareness may result; in the worst-case scenario, where the pressure from the high oxygen flow is transmitted directly to the lungs, severe barotrauma can occur. Modern machines address this problem by having oxygen flushes which cannot be accidentally left on.

Carbon dioxide is sometimes used to stimulate ventilation at the end of an operation, and accidents have occurred when the anaesthetist has forgotten to turn it off before starting the next case. Nowadays, carbon dioxide flowmeters have a low maximum flow setting to minimize the risk of serious consequences to the patient if this happens.

Checking the Machine

It is essential that anaesthetic machines undergo a 'pre-flight check' before an operating list, and it is an unwise anaesthetist who leaves this most important task to his assistant. Checking routines are well established and are designed to work with almost any machine. The checks are mainly designed to confirm the integrity of the oxygen and nitrous oxide supplies and that backups are available, ensure that there are no major leaks, check that the correct vaporizer is properly fitted and filled, and test the breathing system, suction and ventilator for faults. A check list based on that recommended by the Association of Anaesthetists of Great Britain and Ireland can be seen in Figure 4.3.

Breathing Systems

Delivery of the anaesthetic gases from machine to patient is via the breathing system, sometimes known as the circuit. There are different systems for different functions, and the anaesthetist must have an in-depth knowledge of the properties of each system in order to be able to choose the right one for the job and to set the flow rates so that rebreathing of expired carbon dioxide does not occur. It will suffice here to describe a few of the basic systems and highlight their features.

Lack

The Lack system has largely taken over from its predecessor, the Magill, as the position of the expiratory valve on the latter made scavenging difficult (see below). It is ideal for the spontaneously breathing adult, but is notoriously inefficient (i.e. causes marked rebreathing of carbon dioxide) if the lungs are ventilated artificially. The diagram below (Figure 4.4A) shows the reservoir bag and adjustable pressure-limiting valve ('pop-off' valve) which are common to so many circuits.

Bain

Figure 4.4B shows the parallel, rather than the more common co-axial, form of the Bain system. Although superficially resembling the Lack system, it can be seen that the relationship between the fresh gas flow, the valve and

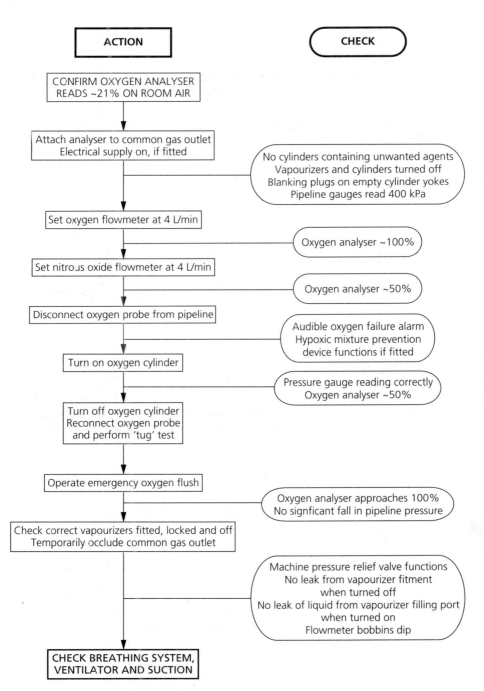

Figure 4.3 A simplified anaesthetic machine check list.

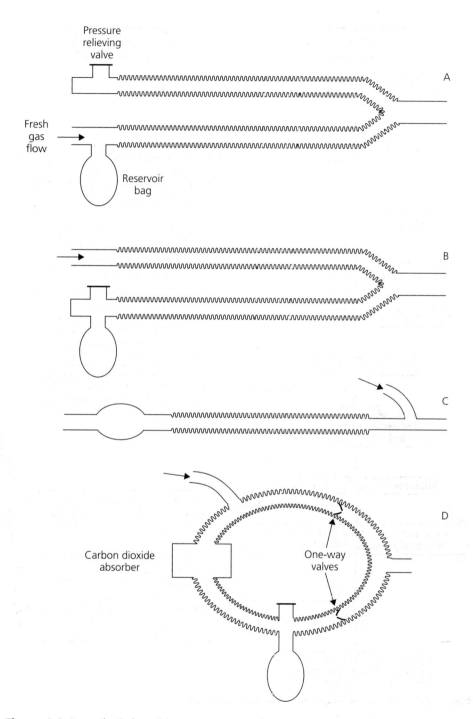

Figure 4.4 Anaesthetic breathing systems. A. Lack; B. Bain; C. Ayre's T-piece with Jackson–Rees bag; D. Circle system.

the bag differs, and this change is enough to reverse completely the properties of the system, which is good for positive-pressure ventilation but inefficient for spontaneous breathing.

T-piece

Although not looking much like it, the T-piece (here modified by the addition of an open-ended reservoir bag) behaves in a similar manner to the Bain system (Figure 4.4C). The T-piece is commonly used for small children, when the low internal volume and lack of a pressure-relieving valve confer a significant advantage.

Circle

A quick glance at Figure 4.4D and Figure 4.5 will show that the circle system is considerably more complex than the others. It is really in a different

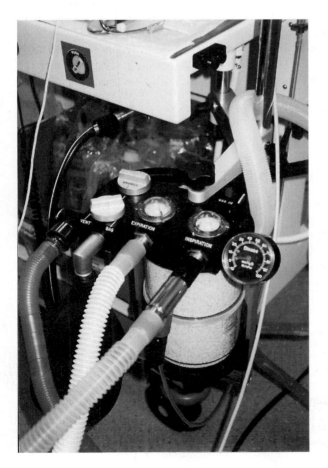

Figure 4.5 The complexities of the circle system.

category entirely, and allows expired gas to be reused by the patient by passing it through a chemical (soda-lime) which absorbs carbon dioxide. Two one-way valves direct gas around the circle, thus ensuring that there is no risk of breathing a mixture from which carbon dioxide has not been removed. The circle is a very versatile piece of equipment and can be used with very low fresh gas flows, thus reducing atmospheric pollution (see below) and saving money on the cost of expensive volatile agents. However, its complexity means that oxygen and carbon dioxide monitoring are essential and that monitoring of the concentration of volatile agent should accompany the use of low flows (Figure 4.5).

Scavenging

The evidence linking chronic exposure to low levels of anaesthetic agents to long-term side-effects is weak, but concerns about the risk of fetal abnormalities and bone marrow depression, amongst others, have led to increasing controls on the levels of these agents in the theatre environment. Recent European legislation under the Control of Substances Hazardous to Health (COSHH) regulations has made strict controls a legal requirement.

The purpose of scavenging is to direct waste anaesthetic gases away from the operating theatre and into the open air where they will disperse. A scavenging tube is attached to the pressure-relieving valve of the breathing system and acts as a conduit for the gases, sometimes assisted by a small negative pressure. Nothing is without its hazards, and accidentally blocked scavenging pipes have led to excessive pressures being applied to patients' lungs with consequent barotrauma.

Ventilators

At its simplest, a ventilator is a device which takes over the work of breathing for a patient. Negative-pressure ventilators, which suck air into the lungs by creating a partial vacuum in a rigid cage enclosing the chest, are still occasionally used for long-term respiratory support, but the vast majority of ventilators are positive-pressure, blowing gas into the lungs, and it is these which will be discussed here.

Types of Ventilator

There are many different (and confusing) ways of classifying mechanical ventilators, but a functional classification into two groups is the most useful.

MINUTE-VOLUME DIVIDERS
As exemplified by the Manley ventilator (Figure 4.6), the main work-horse of British anaesthesia, these machines work by taking the continuous flow

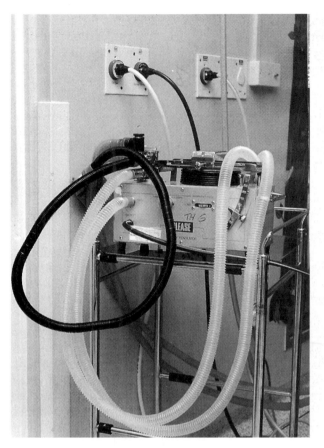

Figure 4.6 Manley ventilator—a minute-volume divider.

of fresh gas from the anaesthetic machine (the minute volume) and dividing it into a fixed number (frequency) of tidal breaths per minute. The ventilator is powered by the fresh gas supply itself, and is a simple and robust machine which can cope with most situations.

'BAG SQUEEZERS'

As their name suggests, these ventilators take the place of the anaesthetist's hand which squeezes the reservoir bag manually to ventilate a patient's lungs (Figure 4.7). As such, they can be used with any breathing system suitable for positive-pressure ventilation such as the Bain, T-piece or circle. They tend to be more complex than the minute-volume dividers and more versatile, as minute volume, tidal volume and frequency can all be set independently of the fresh gas flow. Since these ventilators are not directly interposed in the fresh gas flow they need a separate power supply, usually either an independent compressed gas source or electricity.

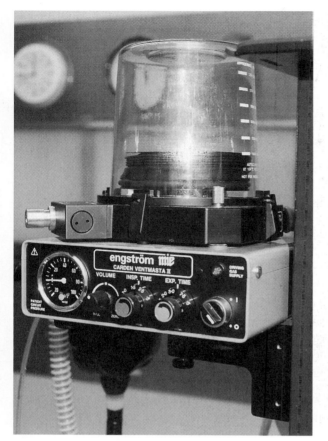

Figure 4.7 Carden ventilator—a 'bag squeezer' ventilator.

Features of Ventilators

The simplest ventilator, such as the Manley, has controls for adjusting the tidal volume/frequency, the pressure generated during inspiration and the inspiratory/expiratory time ratio. More complex machines, especially those used in intensive care, have a variety of other features, such as:

- Alarms to alert the operator to disconnection, high airway pressures, etc.
- Positive end-expiratory pressure control to enable the patient to breathe out against a resistance, thus splinting open the alveoli and improving oxygenation.
- Synchronization of positive-pressure breaths with the patient's own respiratory attempts.
- A facility which allows the patient to breathe spontaneously and only provides an artificial breath if the minute volume falls below a pre-set value. Both of the above help to 'wean' patients off the ventilator as they are recovering.

- A 'sigh' function which helps to prevent alveolar collapse (atelectasis) by providing occasional large tidal-volume breaths.
- A selection of different inspiratory waveforms to suit patients with diseases such as asthma, adult respiratory distress syndrome (ARDS), etc.

Maintenance of the Airway

Maintaining a clear passage for inspiratory and expiratory gas in the unconscious patient is one of the most important tasks for the anaesthetist and a variety of tools exist to help. Airway obstruction largely occurs because of the tendency of the tongue to 'fall back' in the unconscious patient, coming into direct contact with the posterior pharyngeal wall and preventing free passage of air from the mouth or nose into the trachea.

Face Mask

When used properly, a face mask ensures an air-tight fit between the patient's face and the breathing system, thus limiting pollution of the theatre environment and preventing the entrainment of room air into the anaesthetic gases breathed by the patient (Figure 4.8). Face masks are usually made of black rubber, but there has been a recent trend towards using clear plastic; this has the double advantage of allowing the anaesthetist to see any regurgitated gastric contents before they slip down the trachea, and of being less frightening for the patient who is being given oxygen before induction.

Airways

The airway is inserted over the tongue to bring it forward off the posterior pharyngeal wall, and is often used in conjunction with the face mask. Hard plastic oral, or soft rubber nasal versions are available in different sizes (Figure 4.8). The correct use of the airway can relieve a totally obstructed patient rapidly, but it is important not to insert it when the patient is only lightly anaesthetized, as coughing, laryngospasm, retching and vomiting can all be induced by the stimulation of the uvula.

Tracheal Tubes

Invented by Ivan Magill in 1920 (and rejected as being of 'no practical use' by his PhD assessors), the tracheal tube is still the gold standard against which other methods of airway control are compared. Passed nasally or orally into the trachea, the tube almost guarantees a clear airway, allows access for suction or lavage, protects the lungs from regurgitated gastric contents and, most importantly, allows the use of positive-pressure ventilation without any risk of gastric distension. Reusable rubber tubes have

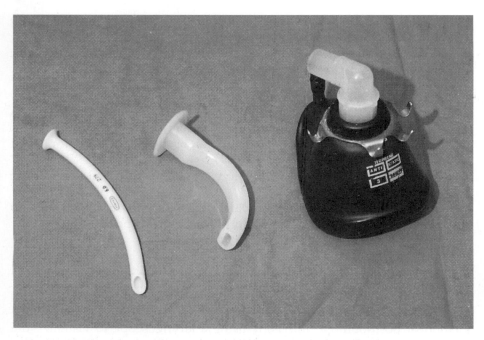

Figure 4.8 Airway maintenance equipment. From left: nasal airway, oral airway, face mask.

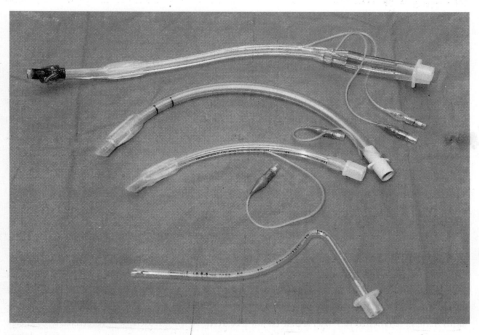

Figure 4.9 Tracheal tubes. From top: double-lumen endobronchial tube, armoured tube, standard oral tracheal tube, pre-formed nasal tube.

largely been superseded by disposable PVC tubes, and these are available in a variety of styles for different purposes, some of which are illustrated in Figure 4.9:

- The standard cuffed tube – the cuff is inflated in the trachea to provide an air-tight seal and completely protect the trachea from gastric contents.
- The uncuffed tube – used in children because the cuff can result in ischaemia and oedema of the tracheal mucosa.
- The pre-formed tube – available in oral or nasal versions for facial surgery.
- The double-lumen tube – for isolation or ventilation of one lung during thoracic surgery.
- The armoured tube – resistant to kinking, and used when the head is to be manipulated or the patient is to lie in the prone position.

The Laryngoscope

Although Magill described passage of the tracheal tube blindly through the nose, and this technique is still sometimes used today, the standard method of positioning a tube is by using a laryngoscope to visualize the laryngeal inlet. The Macintosh laryngoscope, designed in 1943, has withstood the test of time and remains the most popular model, but there are as many different laryngoscope styles as anaesthetists who want their names immortalized, and some of the more important ones are illustrated in Figure 4.10:

- The Macintosh – with the trademark curved blade designed to fit between the vallecula and the epiglottis.
- The Magill – straight-bladed to pass over the epiglottis.
- The Seward – one of many styles designed to facilitate intubation in children.
- The McCoy – a modified Macintosh with a levering tip to aid in difficult intubation.
- The fibreoptic intubating scope – a flexible fibreoptic instrument for difficult intubation.

The Laryngeal Mask Airway

No discussion of modern airway management would be complete without mention of the laryngeal mask airway (LMA) designed and introduced by Archie Brain in the 1980s. One of the few major advances in anaesthetic practice in recent years, the LMA is a cross between an oral airway and a face mask (Figure 4.11). Inserted blindly into a well-anaesthetized patient and with the cuff inflated, the 'bowl' of the LMA sits snugly over the laryngeal inlet, and allows the patient to breathe spontaneously with no obstruction, while relieving the anaesthetist from the tiring and often painful chore of maintaining a clear airway with a mask and a strong right hand. Without

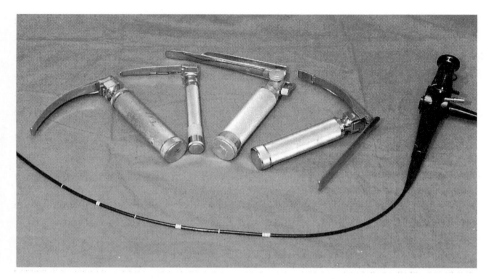

Figure 4.10 Layrngoscopes. From left: Macintosh, Seward, Magill, McCoy. The fibre-optic scope lies underneath.

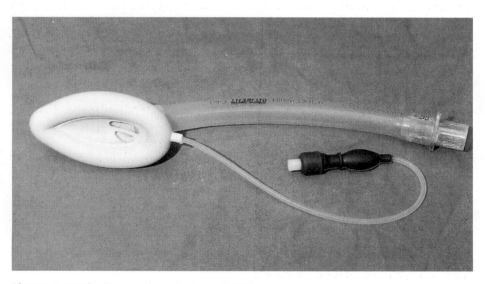

Figure 4.11 The laryngeal mask airway (LMA).

this disincentive, anaesthetists are rediscovering anaesthesia without muscle relaxation, which may well be a considerable contribution to patient safety. The LMA can be tolerated during recovery until very light levels of anaes-thesia, and a clear airway can therefore be anticipated until the patient is sufficiently awake to manage their own reflexes. The extended role of the LMA now includes its use in place of a tracheal tube in certain categories of ventilated patients.

Key Points

- Modern anaesthesia relies on the availability of sophisticated equipment.

- Patient safety is the foremost concern when designing and using anaesthetic equipment.

- It is mandatory to perform safety checks before using an anaesthetic machine.

- Scavenging apparatus is an essential part of the anaesthetic machine to protect personnel from the possible harmful effects of chronic exposure to gases.

- The laryngeal mask airway (LMA) is an important development in airway maintenance in the unconscious patient.

Further Reading

Davey, A., Moyle, J.T.B., Ward, C.S. 1992: *Ward's anaesthetic equipment*. London: WB Saunders.

Parbook, G.D., Davies, P.D., Parbook, E.O. *Basic physics and measurement in Anaesthesia*. London: Heinemann.

Monitoring

5

Introduction

The nineteenth-century French physiologist Claude Bernard wrote 'Only within very narrow boundaries can man observe the phenomena which surround him. . . . To extend his knowledge, he has had to increase the power of his organs by means of special appliances.' This emphasizes an important aspect of modern anaesthetic monitoring, which is that the machines do not *replace* the observations of the anaesthetist, but extend their range and sometimes increase their accuracy. These machines may also free the hands of the anaesthetist for other important tasks (maintaining the airway, preparing drugs, etc.) and may be the only way of observing inaccessible patients (for example, during radiotherapy). In addition, alarms help vigilance during long or complicated cases.

Various anaesthetic organizations around the world have published recommended standards of monitoring, and it is no surprise that they all emphasize the great importance of the continued presence of the anaesthetist in the operating room at all times. The anaesthetist may detect a change (or the potential for change) before the monitoring machine does or before the alarm sounds, and of course the anaesthetist needs to be present to respond appropriately to a change detected by the monitors.

It must also be remembered that all monitoring devices have their limitations and drawbacks. Any monitor can give misleading information in some circumstances, and even non-invasive monitoring can cause harm to the patient – for example, by the effects of pressure or by electrical damage. Generally, of course, the risk/benefit balance is greatly in favour of the extensive use of monitoring, and this has even been recognized by the insurance industry – anaesthetists in Massachusetts pay lower malpractice premiums if they adopt the local minimum monitoring standards.

Monitoring of the Circulation

Monitoring by the Anaesthetist

The anaesthetist may obtain direct information about the circulation by palpation of the pulse, observation of peripheral perfusion, and sometimes by using a precordial or oesophageal stethoscope. Further information can be gained by observation of blood loss and urine output (in the catheterized patient). Both the patient and the surgeon must be observed for signs of unexpected bleeding. Blood loss may be obvious visually, and the patient may become hypotensive, tachycardic and vasoconstricted. Depending on the surgeon, other signs may be shouting, muttering or total silence, but the cardinal sign is the absence of chatter about golf or the stock market! The enlightened surgeon will calmly announce 'This tumour seems to be stuck to the aorta but I'm sure I can dissect it out'. Any of these signs will give more time to make preparations for massive blood transfusion.

Monitoring by Machines

Blood pressure is the most easily measured index of the adequacy of the circulation. The classic mercury manometer is too cumbersome for use during surgery, but other machines are available. Manual devices such as the oscillotonometer have largely been superseded by electrically powered, automatic machines, but still have a place. Both the manual and the automatic devices work on the same principle as the mercury manometer, which is familiar to all medical students. As the pressure within the cuff is gradually reduced, systolic pressure is detected by the presence of turbulence in the artery, and this turbulence is detected by a stethoscope (classic technique), by a second cuff connected to an oscillating needle (oscillotonometer), or by a pressure detector attached to the cuff (many automatic machines). Diastolic pressure is detected in an analogous fashion.

For very major surgery or in patients with severe cardiac disease, direct intra-arterial blood pressure monitoring is often used. This involves the insertion of a cannula into a peripheral artery (commonly the radial) and the use of a 'transducer' (a device which converts one form of energy into another) to convert the pressure signal into electrical energy. The systolic and diastolic pressures are shown on a screen, along with the waveform, which can give additional information. Drawbacks of the use of intra-arterial monitoring include subsequent occlusion of the artery and the potential for accidental intra-arterial injection of drugs, which may cause severe limb ischaemia. Figure 5.1 shows a cannula in a radial artery with manometer tubing leading to a transducer (arrow), and Figure 5.2 shows the resulting waveform (bottom trace).

Sometimes it is necessary to gain an accurate idea of the adequacy of the circulating volume, particularly during major cases. A central venous pressure monitor can then be used and gives information on the filling pressure of the right side of the heart. A long cannula is inserted into a central vein (usually the internal jugular but sometimes the subclavian) and is then connected to a saline manometer; when the manometer is connected to the cannula, the pressure in the superior vena cava is the same as that in the manometer and can easily be read (see Figure 5.3). A zero reference point must always be used and quoted when measuring central venous pressure – commonly this is the mid-axillary line or the sternal angle. Central venous

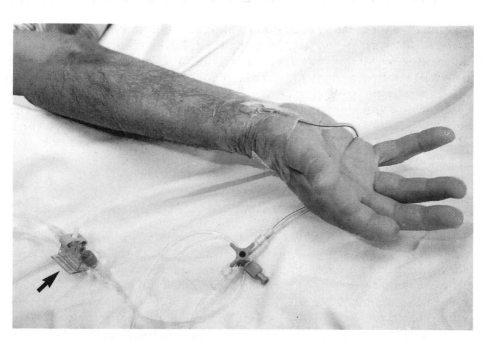

Figure 5.1 Cannula in a radial artery with manometer tubing leading to a transducer (arrowed).

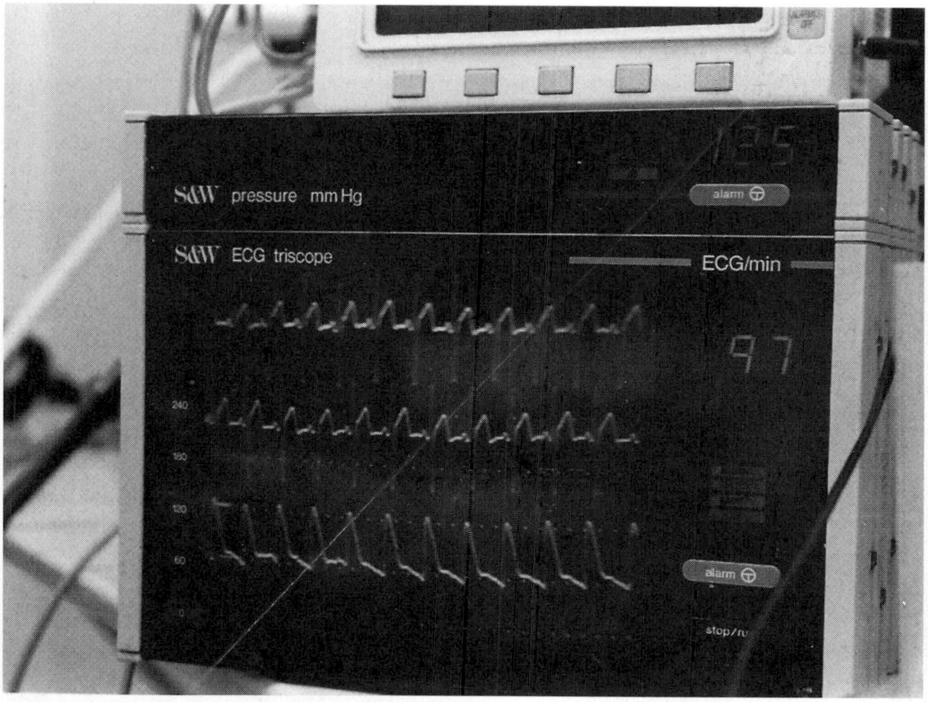

Figure 5.2 Arterial pressure waveform (bottom trace) recorded from the system shown in Figure 5.1.

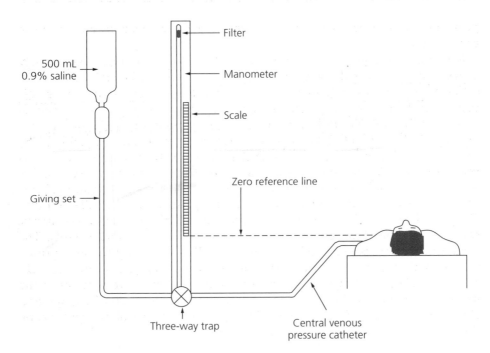

Figure 5.3 The saline manometer as used to monitor central venous pressure (CVP).

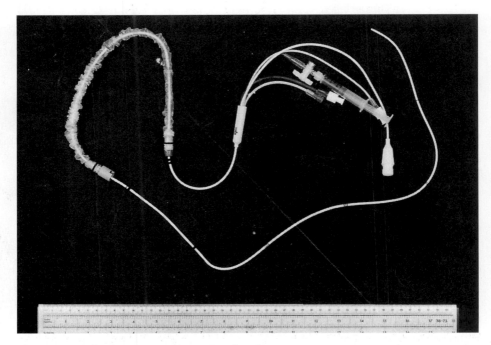

Figure 5.4 Pulmonary artery (Swan–Ganz) catheter.

pressure can also be measured by connecting the catheter to an electronic transducer.

For more accurate assessment of the state of the circulation, particularly in intensive care, a balloon-tipped pulmonary artery catheter ('Swan-Ganz' catheter) is often used (Figure 5.4). This is a longer version of the central venous pressure cannula with an inflatable balloon on the end, and is advanced through the right atrium and right ventricle into the pulmonary artery until the inflated balloon 'wedges' in a pulmonary arteriole. The pressure transmitted up the lumen of the catheter is then pulmonary venous pressure and, since there are no valves in the pulmonary venous system, this is equivalent to left atrial pressure. By Starling's Law, the circulating volume can be increased until the left atrial pressure gives optimal cardiac output. Figure 5.5 shows the pressure measured through the pulmonary artery catheter as it is advanced through the various chambers and vessels. The same device can also be used to measure cardiac output by the Fick principle. A small volume (usually 10 mL) of cold saline is injected into the right atrium and the resulting temperature change measured by a monitor in the distal part of the catheter in the pulmonary artery; the rate of change and absolute change in temperature are determined by the cardiac output, i.e. by the amount of blood flowing through the heart.

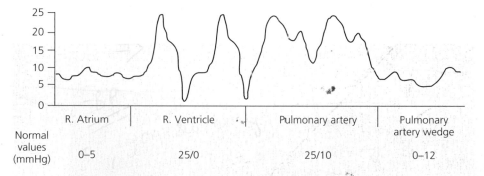

Figure 5.5 Pressure changes recorded from a Swan–Ganz catheter as it is advanced from the superior vena cava to a branch of the pulmonary artery.

An approximation to cardiac output can be obtained by advancing an echocardiography probe into the oesophagus and obtaining echocardiographic representations of the dimensions of the left ventricle. At the moment this is of limited clinical use.

It is usual to monitor the electrocardiogram during every anaesthetic. This is most useful for following changes in rate and rhythm. Since only one lead can be displayed at a time, its usefulness for detecting myocardial ischaemia is limited, unless the changes are gross.

Monitoring of the Respiratory System

Monitoring by the Anaesthetist

Hypoxia may be detected by the appearance of cyanosis in the patient. Clinical cyanosis requires the presence of 4–5 g/dL of reduced haemoglobin, so the sign may not be present in a grossly anaemic patient who becomes hypoxic. Clinical signs related to ventilation include the adequacy and pattern of chest movement, and auscultation of the lung fields. The latter sign is most important immediately after intubation, when it is essential to check that the tracheal tube is in the trachea and not the oesophagus, and that both lung fields are ventilated equally to ensure that the tube has not been passed down into the right main bronchus.

Monitoring by Machine

Continuous, accurate measurement of the adequacy of oxygenation of the blood is now possible using the pulse oximeter (Figure 5.6). This device measures the percentage of haemoglobin which is in the oxygenated form, by shining light of two wavelengths through tissue. The two wavelengths are absorbed to different degrees by oxygenated and de-oxygenated haemoglobin, so measurement of the absorption gives the proportion of the two

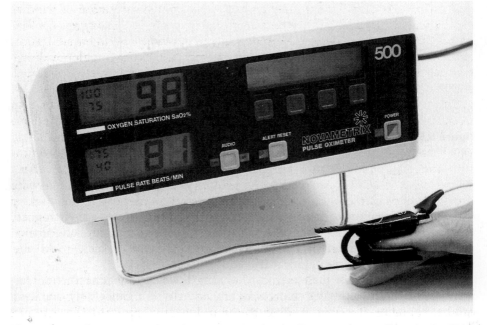

Figure 5.6 Pulse oximeter showing probe on subject's finger and recording obtained.

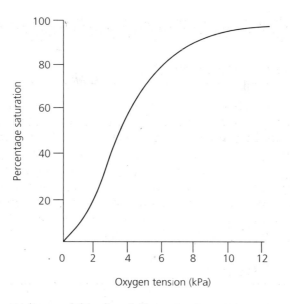

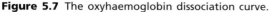

Figure 5.7 The oxyhaemoglobin dissociation curve.

forms of haemoglobin. Normally this would include the haemoglobin in both arterial and venous blood, but of course we are only interested in that in arterial blood. Consequently, the pulse oximeter isolates the pulsatile component of the signal so that the displayed saturation is that in arterial blood only.

The oximeter signal, of course, gives the percentage saturation of haemoglobin with oxygen. What we would prefer to know is the oxygen content or partial pressure. There is a predictable relationship between saturation and partial pressure which is given by the familiar oxyhaemoglobin dissociation curve (Figure 5.7). It is obvious from the approximately sigmoid shape of the curve that there can be quite a large fall in partial pressure before the saturation changes very much, so that apparently minor changes in saturation at the upper end of the curve may have quite profound effects on oxygen partial pressure. It is worth emphasizing that a saturation below about 91–92 per cent is regarded as being clinically important, while clinical recognition of cyanosis cannot occur until the saturation falls below about 75 per cent, which represents a quite profound degree of hypoxia. Despite the limitations of measurement of oxygen saturation, there is no satisfactory method of continuous, non-invasive monitoring of arterial partial pressure of oxygen, and the pulse oximeter has become an invaluable monitor of oxygenation during anaesthesia, in the early post-operative period and in the intensive care unit.

Oxygenation is only one aspect of respiratory function. Carbon dioxide must be eliminated, and monitoring of arterial carbon dioxide concentration is also valuable. Due to the rapid equilibration of carbon dioxide between blood and alveolar gas, analysis of alveolar gas gives an approximation to

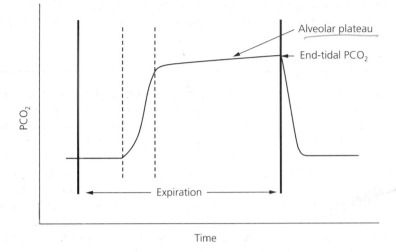

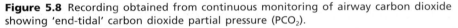

Figure 5.8 Recording obtained from continuous monitoring of airway carbon dioxide showing 'end-tidal' carbon dioxide partial pressure (PCO_2).

the carbon dioxide content of arterial blood. We can monitor alveolar gas by monitoring the composition of the last part of each exhalation – the carbon dioxide content normally reaches a 'plateau' which corresponds to the concentration in alveolar gas (Figure 5.8). The analysis of carbon dioxide is usually carried out by infrared absorption spectrometry.

Both pulse oximetry and capnography (measurement of expired carbon dioxide concentration) suffer from various limitations and inaccuracies. For accurate work, such as major surgery in high-risk patients or in intensive care, it is necessary to measure the partial pressures of oxygen and carbon dioxide in arterial blood directly, by taking a sample of arterial blood (often from an arterial line) and exposing it to an oxygen electrode and a carbon dioxide electrode in a 'blood gas analyser'. This machine also measures pH and bicarbonate concentration and thereby gives information on the degree of metabolic acid–base disturbance as well as the respiratory disturbance, which is derived from the carbon dioxide partial pressure.

Monitoring of the Neurological and Neuromuscular Systems

Monitoring by the Anaesthetist

The depth of anaesthesia and the degree of neuromuscular relaxation may be assessed in a gross fashion by looking for movement, tensing of the abdominal muscles, lacrimation, sweating and so on. In the neurosurgical patient, or the head-injured patient on the ward or intensive care unit, the clinical signs of raised intracranial pressure are also important. Pupillary size, heart rate, vomiting, and degree of spontaneous movement should all be assessed at regular intervals together with an assessment of level of consciousness.

Monitoring by Machine

Unfortunately there is no reliable way of monitoring depth of anaesthesia. Indirect signs such as the clinical signs mentioned above, plus blood pressure, heart rate and the presence of arrhythmias may all give a rough guide but can be affected by many other factors. Techniques based on the electroencephalogram (EEG) have been tried: these include the cerebral function monitor (CFM), cerebral function analysis monitor (CFAM) and spectral edge analysis, all of which have been found wanting. The evoked response of a specific area of sensory cortex may be more promising in some situations: auditory evoked potentials, somatosensory evoked potentials and visual evoked potentials all have applications but none is specific enough to be used routinely as a general monitor of anaesthetic depth.

Clinical monitoring of intracranial pressure (ICP) has been mentioned above. In the patient with a severe head injury or certain neurosurgical patients, it may be preferable to measure ICP directly. The pressure may be measured from within the cerebral ventricle, the subdural space or the extradural space. All these approaches require a minor neurosurgical operation and are not undertaken lightly, but do give invaluable information especially when ICP is changing rapidly.

The peripheral nerve stimulator is an important, if not essential, monitor whenever muscle relaxants are being used (see Chapter 3). It monitors neuromuscular function and enables the anaesthetist to assess the depth of muscle relaxation during surgery without having to rely on subjective impressions. Just as importantly, it is used to confirm that the effect of the muscle relaxant has worn off or been reversed by an anticholinesterase before the trachea is extubated and the patient taken to the recovery room. The details of the peripheral nerve stimulator are beyond the scope of this book, but its use involves the application of an electrical current transcutaneously over a convenient nerve and observation of the resulting response in the muscle. Convenient nerves include the facial nerve and the ulnar nerve at the wrist.

Monitoring of Blood Chemistry and Other Variables

This almost invariably needs to be done by machine. Changes in acid–base status, electrolytes and/or blood sugar concentrations may be heralded by clinical changes such as tachycardia or arrhythmias but always need confirmation by measurement of a blood sample. Blood sugar is conveniently estimated in the operating theatre by colorimetric techniques such as 'BM-stix' without having to bother the clinical chemistry laboratory. Acid–base status and electrolyte estimation take just a few minutes with modern machines, and it may well take longer to telephone the laboratory and transport the specimen than to perform the measurement itself. Consequently, there is increasing availability of acid–base machines and sodium/potassium electrodes in intensive care units and operating suites.

The haematology laboratory may also become involved in monitoring for the anaesthetist. Following a massive blood transfusion, clotting may be impaired because of the absence of many clotting factors from stored blood. Clotting problems are often clinically obvious and are clearly recognized as severe when incision sites and venepuncture sites start to ooze again after having clotted. Most blood banks are reluctant to issue fresh frozen plasma, platelet concentrate and clotting factors on the basis of a clinical impression, and a clotting screen is usually required. Many an anaesthetist has become apoplectic when expected to leave a patient who appears to be exsanguinating in order to discuss the finer points of the clotting cascade with the haematology laboratory. A telephone call at the end of the case to thank the haematology department for their assistance ('we couldn't have managed without your help') normally restores friendly relations.

Monitoring of the Anaesthetic Machine

Monitoring by the Anaesthetist

The proper functioning of the anaesthetic machine is a vital part of delivering a safe anaesthetic (see Chapter 4). Checking the machine before the start of the list has become as integral a part of the anaesthetist's activities as the pre-operative visit to the patient.

It is essential to continue regular observation of the machine during the anaesthetic. Flowmeters must be inspected to make sure that a hypoxic mixture is not being delivered, the vaporizers must be inspected and refilled if appropriate, and the breathing system must be inspected to make sure that the ventilator is working properly and that there has been no disconnection. Many of these can be 'observed' continuously by listening for auditory cues – for example, a change in the rhythm of the ventilator or a change in the note of the expiratory valve. Anaesthetists may therefore be sensitive about extraneous noise in the theatre, such as loud conversation or accompanying music. There is rarely an objection to background music, and a calm surgeon is a small price to pay for idiosyncratic musical taste, but 'background' music may become 'foreground' music and then interfere with the anaesthetist's monitoring activities.

Monitoring by Machine

Virtually anything the machine does can now be monitored. The inspired oxygen concentration should always be measured (by paramagnetic oxygen sensor or fuel cell), and often the inspired concentrations of nitrous oxide and volatile agent (by infrared absorption spectrometry). Measurement of inspired and expired tidal volume and minute volume help to identify changes before identifiable problems of hypoxia or hypercapnia occur. Measurement of the pressure in the ventilator helps to identify circuit disconnections at an early stage, and also shows when the inflation pressure is rising (as may happen, for example, if the tracheal tube is kinked, if bronchospasm occurs or if there is a tension pneumothorax).

Alarms

The use and abuse of monitor alarms is a subject in its own right. The anaesthetist's vigilance needs to be applied to so many variables at the same time that alarms are essential to attract his attention immediately to something which has gone beyond acceptable limits. If alarms are too sensitive, however, they may be counter-productive. A variety of penetrating noises occurring at frequent intervals is irritating and upsetting to all present. It is generally in the patient's interests that surgery proceeds in a calm and relaxed atmosphere, so unnecessary irritations should be avoided.

Instrument manufacturers are devoting significant time and money to the psychology of alarms. Alarms should attract attention without being constantly irritating, and it should be easy to distinguish between alarms relating to different systems.

Key Points

- Despite the existence of machines to monitor many variables, clinical monitoring by the anaesthetist remains essential.
- It is generally accepted that the use of certain 'minimal monitoring' standards improves patient safety.
- All monitors have a risk/benefit ratio. 'The more, the better' is not necessarily true.
- Monitors have to be interpreted intelligently and acted upon.

Further Reading

Davey, A.J., Moyle, J.T.B., Ward, C.S. 1992: *Ward's anaesthetic equipment*. London: WB Saunders.

PART TWO

The Anaesthetist Outside the Operating Theatre

Pre-operative Preparation

6

Introduction

The primary aim of the anaesthetist's pre-operative visit is to ensure that the patient is presented for theatre in an optimal state, so that the risks of anaesthesia and surgery are reduced to a minimum. Additionally, it offers an opportunity to discuss options with the patient (for example, general versus regional anaesthesia, or techniques of post-operative analgesia), to plan the anaesthetic and, of course, to prescribe premedication if appropriate. Patients are almost invariably anxious about anaesthesia; typical worries include awareness, 'not waking up', post-operative pain and the revealing of indiscretions whilst under the anaesthetic (in fact, an extremely rare phenomenon). Appropriate reassurance may be offered in relation to all of these anxieties: awareness and 'not waking up' are both extremely rare, post-operative pain is receiving increasing attention, and no anaesthetist has ever become rich by being privy to the secrets of company directors or government ministers!

With modern anaesthetic techniques, it is extremely unusual for a patient to be labelled 'unfit for anaesthesia'. Rather, the less fit patient may have his operation delayed in order to improve his general medical condition, and possibly to facilitate more invasive and elaborate monitoring in theatre. A period of recovery in an intensive care unit or high–dependency unit may also be planned, depending on the length, extent and invasiveness of the proposed operation. It follows that the anaesthetist's visit must be early enough to modify or initiate therapy and to make appropriate post-operative arrangements.

Anaesthesia may be influenced by any physiological system so each of these needs to be considered in turn.

Patient Assessment

The Cardiovascular System

CORONARY ARTERY DISEASE

- It is important to establish the severity of this common condition. Exercise tolerance is the simplest indication, and has the advantage that the physiological changes associated with exercise are similar to those associated with surgery, particularly in terms of the extra demand placed on the heart. Other useful information includes frequency of angina (including any recent change), drug consumption and number of hospital admissions. A particular problem occurs with patients who have had a myocardial infarction within the preceding six months: such patients have a significantly increased risk of reinfarction and death in the post-operative period, so all but the most urgent surgery should be delayed until at least six months after myocardial infarction.

Patients with stable, well-controlled angina usually present little problem but those with unstable or poorly controlled disease may benefit from a period of treatment with, for example, a beta-blocker or calcium antagonist before surgery is undertaken.

CARDIAC FAILURE

This should be controlled before surgery, especially if associated with physical signs such as basal crepitations or gallop rhythm. Exercise tolerance again gives useful information about the severity of the disease.

Diuretics remain the mainstay of treatment, but care must be taken not to cause dehydration or electrolyte imbalance.

ARRHYTHMIAS

These can only be diagnosed accurately from the electrocardiogram (see below), although the patient may give a history of palpitations or Stokes–Adams attacks, or an irregular pulse may be felt. Infrequent ectopic beats are rarely significant unless they are secondary to, for example, electrolyte imbalance or thyroid disease. Other arrhythmias may require control before surgery; atrial fibrillation requires treatment with digoxin, especially if the rate is fast, while heart block usually requires insertion of a temporary or permanent pacemaker.

HYPERTENSION

Patients commonly arrive on the surgical ward with a blood pressure within the hypertensive range. Considering the stresses associated with admission to hospital, this is not surprising, and in most of these patients, blood pressure reverts to normal over the next 12–24 hours. The risks of anaesthesia and surgery are known to be increased when the diastolic blood pressure persistently exceeds 110 mmHg; in particular, there is a higher risk of stroke and myocardial infarction. All such patients should have blood pressure controlled before surgery, as should patients with slightly lower blood pressure but significant end-organ damage (left ventricular hypertrophy, renal impairment or previous stroke). Patients who are already receiving antihypertensive treatment but still have abnormally high blood pressure may require additional treatment or a change in existing treatment. **All patients receiving antihypertensive drugs should continue treatment up to and including the day of surgery.**

The Respiratory System

THE UPPER AIRWAY

This may be considered to extend from the lips to the trachea. A few patients present with conditions, such as tumours of the mouth or pharynx, which may completely obstruct the upper airway during anaesthesia. Special care and special techniques are required during induction of anaesthesia, and these patients require detailed assessment by the anaesthetist.

CHRONIC OBSTRUCTIVE AIRWAYS DISEASE (INCLUDING ASTHMA)

The severity of this condition is most easily assessed by reference to the patient's exercise tolerance, together with drug usage and frequency of related hospital admissions. Physical signs such as cyanosis or wheeze are, of course, important in more severe disease. A chest X-ray rarely helps unless there is a history of recent worsening of symptoms, and the X-ray may then show a localized pneumonia or occasionally a small pneumothorax. More elaborate investigations, such as arterial blood gas measurement and spirometry, may help in selected cases.

Patients with severe obstructive airways disease often benefit from early admission to hospital, so that they may have intensive physiotherapy and regular bronchodilator treatment. Regular measurement of peak expiratory flow rate helps to gauge improvement. Regional techniques are often preferred for these patients; if general anaesthesia is chosen, it is important to avoid drugs which release histamine (for example, thiopentone and d-tubocurarine).

OTHER RESPIRATORY DISEASES

Patients with an acute infection of the upper or lower respiratory tract should have elective surgery deferred until the infection has cleared, otherwise there is a risk of life-threatening respiratory tract infection in the postoperative period. Pneumothoraces (however small) and pleural effusions should be drained before surgery. Other less common conditions such as bronchiectasis, cystic fibrosis and fibrosing alveolitis require liaison between surgeon, physician and anaesthetist in order to select the best timing and preparation for surgery.

The Endocrine System

DIABETES MELLITUS

Diabetic patients have a high incidence of cardiovascular and renal disease and should be assessed accordingly. The most common practical problem with these patients is management of the diabetes during the inevitable period of starvation – which may extend from a few hours if the surgery is minor to several days in the case of extensive intra-abdominal surgery. The diabetes should be reasonably, but not obsessively, controlled beforehand; a random blood sugar below about 15 mmol/L is probably acceptable, and ketonuria should be excluded.

Otherwise, the general principles are as follows:

- Hypoglycaemia *must* be avoided because irreversible brain damage may result.
- Regular measurement of blood sugar concentration is important because any type of surgery may upset the control of even the best-controlled diabetic. Ward measurement using capillary blood and colorimetric sticks such as 'BM-Stix' is usually most convenient, and achieves acceptable accuracy.
- Insulin-dependent diabetics require insulin, even during periods of starvation, to prevent ketosis.
- The hormonal changes associated with surgery (the so-called 'stress response') include release of glucocorticoids, catecholamines and growth hormone, all of which are diabetogenic. It follows that insulin-dependent diabetics may require more insulin than normal, while non-insulin-dependent diabetics may require insulin for a brief period.

A suggested scheme for management of diabetic patients undergoing elective surgery is shown in Table 6.1. Diabetic patients who require emergency surgery are a greater problem, and often require close liaison between surgeon, anaesthetist and physician.

THYROID DISEASE

The patient with uncontrolled hyperthyroidism is at increased risk because any form of surgery may provoke a thyroid crisis, a condition which carries significant morbidity and mortality. At the other extreme, patients with myxoedema may exhibit delayed recovery, hypothermia and cardiac failure.

Table 6.1 Management of the diabetic patient

	Minor surgery	Major surgery[a]
Diet-controlled	Measure blood sugar Rarely require treatment	Measure blood sugar Rarely require insulin
Oral treatment[b]	Measure blood sugar Omit treatment 12–24 hours before surgery	Measure blood sugar Omit treatment 12–24 hours before surgery
	Both groups may require insulin after operation	
Insulin-dependent	Measure blood sugar	Measure blood sugar
	Insulin (injection or infusion)	
	+5% dextrose infusion (together or separately)	

[a]Major surgery may be regarded, as a general guide, as surgery which requires a period of starvation greater than 24 hours.
[b]Oral treatment should be withdrawn at a time appropriate to the duration of action of the agent.

Unfortunately, there is no quick screening test for thyroid function, so assessment of these patients relies on clinical judgment and a high index of suspicion. Elective surgery should be postponed until laboratory tests are complete.

Patients with goitre may have a narrowed or deviated trachea, and X-ray of the thoracic inlet may help to forecast difficulties associated with intubation.

OTHER ENDOCRINE ORGANS

Patients with parathyroid disease present with the problems of hyper- or hypocalcaemia. Disease of the adrenal glands may produce Addison's disease, Conn's syndrome, Cushing's disease or phaeochromocytoma (all rarities). Acromegaly is associated with hypertension, diabetes and difficulty in tracheal intubation. Other endocrine conditions are even rarer, and the interested reader should consult more specialized accounts.

The Neuromuscular System

EPILEPSY

This poses no specific problem for the anaesthetist, beyond the necessity to avoid agents (such as methohexitone, enflurane and possibly propofol) which are suspected of being epileptogenic. It is important that patients receive their usual anticonvulsant treatment on the day of surgery and as soon as possible afterwards.

LOWER MOTOR NEURONE DISEASE

Patients with lower motor neurone disease have an altered response to suxamethonium. Instead of a localized response at the muscle end-plate, there is an immediate response over the entire muscle membrane, releasing large amounts of potassium: this may be enough to cause hyperkalaemic cardiac arrest. Avoidance of suxamethonium is usually not a problem except in the emergency case.

MYASTHENIA GRAVIS

This condition is associated with increased sensitivity to non-depolarizing muscle relaxants, which must therefore be used in extremely small doses, if at all. Patients with severe disease, or those undergoing major surgery, normally require a period of observation or mechanical ventilation on the intensive care unit post-operatively.

MALIGNANT HYPERTHERMIA

This is a rare, familial condition specifically associated with anaesthesia. A hypermetabolic state of skeletal muscle is triggered, usually by volatile agents or suxamethonium, and, if untreated, death almost invariably ensues from the resulting hyperthermia and electrolyte derangements. The mortality is reduced if appropriate treatment is instituted, but it is best to avoid the situation by use of regional techniques or, if general anaesthesia is unavoidable, by use of a vapour-free anaesthetic machine. Susceptible individuals are usually aware of the high mortality, so they will obviously benefit from an early visit by the anaesthetist, and appropriate reassurance.

OTHER MUSCLE DISEASES

There are many types of muscular dystrophy and other muscle diseases, most extremely rare. These conditions require special care in the selection of anaesthetic and muscle relaxant drugs.

STROKE

A patient who has had a previous stroke is at increased risk of a further stroke during periods of haemodynamic instability such as those which may be associated with anaesthesia and surgery. Whilst there is no documented post-stroke 'risk period' in the sense that there is after myocardial infarction (see above), it makes sense not to undertake elective surgery during recovery from a stroke, and to ensure good control of blood pressure if the stroke was associated with hypertension.

The Genito-urinary System

RENAL FAILURE

The pathophysiology of renal failure, whether acute or chronic, is complex. Also relevant are the effects of dialysis, the frequent presence of anaemia and the consequences of the plethora of drugs which these patients may be taking. Anaesthetic considerations include maintenance of fluid and electrolyte balance, and care with the use of drugs which are mainly excreted in urine (principally muscle relaxants). There is often increased sensitivity to the effects of opioid analgesics, and particularly morphine, which has an active metabolite that accumulates in the presence of renal failure.

PREGNANCY

Anaesthesia for elective surgery is usually contraindicated during pregnancy. In early pregnancy there is a risk that anaesthetic agents may be teratogenic, while in later pregnancy premature labour may be precipitated.

The Alimentary System

TEETH

The dislodgement of teeth, caps and crowns during anaesthesia is a common feature of the annual reports of the medical defence organizations and has helped keep many a lawyer in business. It most commonly occurs during a difficult intubation or attempts to maintain a difficult airway. Many patients are quite grateful to be rid of a solitary loose or rotten fang, but damage to expensive dental work usually requires financial recompense from the health authority.

HIATUS HERNIA

This apparently innocuous condition can pose significant problems for the anaesthetist. The incompetence of the lower oesophageal sphincter causes a much greater risk of regurgitation of stomach contents and aspiration into the lungs. It is important to realize that the stomach is never completely empty even after several hours of fasting, so even the 'adequately starved' patient may be at risk.

The risk of regurgitation may be reduced by the use of a rapid-sequence induction (see Chapter 1), and the acidity of the stomach contents reduced by administration of a histamine H_2 antagonist such as cimetidine before surgery.

CIRRHOSIS OF THE LIVER

The main problems are reduced drug metabolism and impaired clotting. Clotting problems are considered later. In anaesthesia, the most important drugs which undergo hepatic metabolism are the opioid analgesics, and these must be prescribed with particular care.

OBESITY

There is an increased incidence of diseases such as coronary artery disease and diabetes mellitus. Airway maintenance, tracheal intubation and ventilation of the lungs are all more difficult than usual. Drug doses are more difficult to calculate since they should be based on lean body mass. Veins are more difficult to find. Simple manoeuvres such as transferring the patient to and from the operating table become fraught with hazard, and many pairs of hands are required; the sight of burly surgeons disappearing for coffee while the petite female anaesthetist transfers the 120 kg patient off the table is not an edifying one!

The Haematological System

CLOTTING DISORDERS

Clotting may be impaired by liver cirrhosis, by drug treatment (for example, warfarin), or by primary haematological disease. If possible, adequate clotting should be ensured before surgery, but this may not be advisable if, for example, the patient is on therapy for a prosthetic heart valve. Treatment to ensure clotting during surgery may need to be continued by the anaesthetist, by administration of, for example, fresh frozen plasma, cryoprecipitate or platelets.

Major regional anaesthetic techniques, particularly epidural and spinal blocks (see Chapter 2), are contraindicated when clotting is impaired, since any accumulation of blood in the vertebral canal may cause pressure damage to nerves.

SICKLE CELL DISEASE

All patients of Afro-Caribbean origin should be screened for the presence of sickle haemoglobin (HbS). Since the gene may also be found in individuals of Mediterranean, Middle Eastern and Indian origin, it may also be appropriate to screen such individuals.

The homozygous patient must be protected as much as possible from factors known to precipitate a crisis. Hydration, warmth, oxygenation, and analgesia must be provided, and there should be close liaison with the haematology department. The heterozygous state rarely presents a problem unless the patient has the rare HbSC genotype or certain types of surgery are proposed (for example, open-heart surgery or surgery using a tourniquet).

The Skeletal System

ARTHRITIS

Arthritis, particularly rheumatoid arthritis, can cause problems to the anaesthetist because of its effects on the neck and jaw. Mouth opening may be limited, and the cervical spine may be either fixed or unstable. The fixed spine may cause intubation to be difficult, and the unstable spine may damage the spinal cord during manipulation of the head. History and physical examination are important, and cervical spine X-rays may reveal instability.

Other affected joints must be protected and supported during surgery. For example, the hip joint may be at risk during attempts to put the patient in the lithotomy position.

Concurrent Drug Treatment

Most drugs which the patient is taking have side-effects which are predictable from a knowledge of their pharmacology. Examples are given in Table 6.2. A few drugs, however, merit special consideration.

MONOAMINE OXIDASE INHIBITORS

These drugs interact with sympathomimetic agents such as ephedrine and certain opioid analgesics to produce a cardiovascular crisis (tachycardia and hypertension) which may be fatal. Unfortunately, it is necessary to discontinue these drugs six weeks before surgery to eliminate this risk, and this is rarely practical. Anaesthesia is safe provided that sympathomimetics are avoided; opioids other than pethidine are believed to be safe.

Table 6.2 Drug interactions in anaesthesia

Drug	Effect
1. CVS	
(i) Potent antihypertensives e.g. beta-blockers, ACE inhibitors	Enhanced hypotensive effect of general or regional anaesthesia
(ii) Anti-arrhythmics e.g. amiodarone, digoxin	Increased risk of bradycardia ± significant myocardial depression. Digoxin may predispose to ventricular arrhythmias
(iii) Diuretics e.g. thiazides, spironolactone	Dehydration and/or electrolyte imbalance
(iv) Sympathomimetics	Increased likelihood of arrhythmias, especially with halothane
(v) Anticoagulants e.g. warfarin	Major regional blocks contraindicated
2. Respiratory system	
(i) Bronchodilators e.g. aminophylline	Increased likelihood of arrhythmias
3. Central nervous system	
(i) Sedatives and hypnotics	Chronic use induces tolerance to effects of general anaesthetics
(ii) Lithium	Enhanced effect of muscle relaxants: polyuria causing dehydration and electrolyte imbalance
(iii) Antidepressants	
tricyclic	Increased risk of arrhythmias
MAOIs	See text
(iv) Antiparkinson drugs	Levodopa increases risk of arrhythmias
(v) Anti-epileptics	Tolerance to effects of general anaesthetics
4. Antimicrobial	Aminoglycosides in high doses enhance effects of muscle relaxants
5. Drugs of abuse	
(i) Tobacco	(a) Reduces O_2 carriage by formation of COHb (b) Chronic use is a major factor in COAD (c) May induce tolerance to anaesthetic effects
(ii) Alcohol	(a) Tolerance to anaesthetics (b) Heavier use may cause liver damage and cardiomyopathy
(iii) Intravenous drug abuse	(a) Tolerance to effects of opioids (b) Risk of hepatitis and AIDS (c) May have difficult veins
6. Hormones and related drugs	
(i) Glucocorticoids	See text
(ii) OCP	
(iii) Hypoglycaemic drugs	Risk of hypoglycaemia in starved patient

STEROIDS

Treatment with glucocorticoids, whether currently or in the previous six months, impairs the response of the adrenal cortex to physical stress, including surgery. It is necessary to give supplementary steroids following any but the most minor surgery. This is usually done by administration of parenteral hydrocortisone, starting at induction. The exact dose depends on the previous maintenance dose of steroids, duration of treatment, and the condition for which it is being given.

ORAL CONTRACEPTIVE PILL (OCP)

Patients taking any oestrogen-containing OCP are known to be at increased risk of developing deep venous thrombosis and pulmonary embolism following anaesthesia and surgery which is associated with impaired mobility in the post-operative period. Treatment should be discontinued one month before surgery in order to eliminate the risk. If emergency surgery is required, low-dose heparin should be given during the peri-operative period. These precautions are generally unnecessary when minor or intermediate surgery is undertaken. However, varicose vein surgery, lower limb orthopaedic surgery, or the presence of other risk factors for venous thrombosis (such as a previous episode) require the same precautions as those which apply for major surgery. The progesterone-only OCP is associated with no increased risk, and no precautions are necessary.

ASA Grading

Clearly, pre-operative assessment may be complicated. Communication, and patient comparisons, may be assisted by use of a 'shorthand' system such as the American Society of Anesthesiologists' (ASA) grading system. This is set out in Table 6.3. Each patient may be allocated a number between 1 and 5 depending on the severity of their general medical condition, 1 being least severe and 5 most severe. For an emergency case, 'E' is added to the grading. Obviously, grade 1 carries the least risk while grade 5E carries the greatest. An example of patient assessment based on the ASA system is given in Table 6.4.

Table 6.3 The ASA grading system

Grade 1	An otherwise healthy patient
Grade 2	A patient with a disease causing mild to moderate systemic disturbance
Grade 3	A patient with a disease causing severe systemic disturbance
Grade 4	A patient with life-threatening disease
Grade 5	A moribund patient with little chance of survival with or without surgery
Any grade may be supplemented by the letter 'E' in the case of emergency surgery	

Table 6.4 Example of patient assessment based on the ASA system

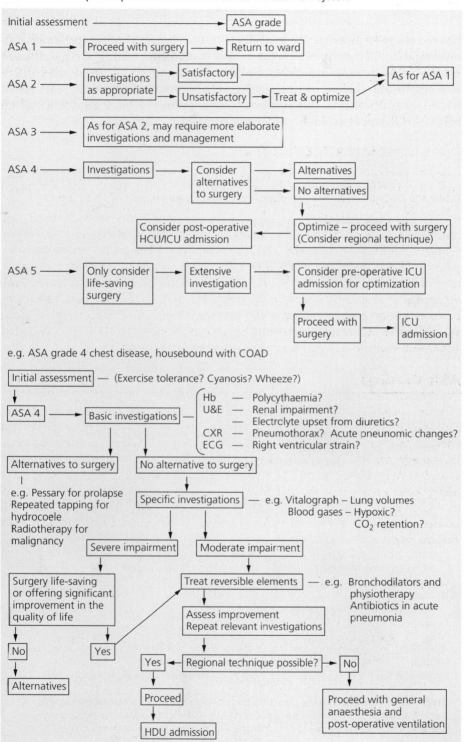

Initial assessment ⟶ ASA grade

ASA 1 ⟶ Proceed with surgery ⟶ Return to ward

ASA 2 ⟶ Investigations as appropriate ⟶ Satisfactory ⟶ As for ASA 1
Investigations as appropriate ⟶ Unsatisfactory ⟶ Treat & optimize ⟶ As for ASA 1

ASA 3 ⟶ As for ASA 2, may require more elaborate investigations and management

ASA 4 ⟶ Investigations ⟶ Consider alternatives to surgery ⟶ Alternatives
Consider alternatives to surgery ⟶ No alternatives ⟶ Optimize – proceed with surgery (Consider regional technique) ⟶ Consider post-operative HCU/ICU admission

ASA 5 ⟶ Only consider life-saving surgery ⟶ Extensive investigation ⟶ Consider pre-operative ICU admission for optimization ⟶ Proceed with surgery ⟶ ICU admission

e.g. ASA grade 4 chest disease, housebound with COAD

Initial assessment — (Exercise tolerance? Cyanosis? Wheeze?)

ASA 4 ⟶ Basic investigations —
Hb — Polycythaemia?
U&E — Renal impairment?
— Electrolyte upset from diuretics?
CXR — Pneumothorax? Acute pneunomic changes?
ECG — Right ventricular strain?

Alternatives to surgery
e.g. Pessary for prolapse
Repeated tapping for hydrocoele
Radiotherapy for malignancy

No alternative to surgery ⟶ Specific investigations — e.g. Vitalograph – Lung volumes
Blood gases – Hypoxic?
CO₂ retention?

Severe impairment ⟶ Surgery life-saving or offering significant improvement in the quality of life ⟶ No ⟶ Alternatives / Yes

Moderate impairment ⟶ Treat reversible elements — e.g. Bronchodilators and physiotherapy Antibiotics in acute pneumonia ⟶ Assess improvement Repeat relevant investigations

Yes ⟵ Regional technique possible? ⟶ No

Yes ⟶ Proceed ⟶ HDU admission

No ⟶ Proceed with general anaesthesia and post-operative ventilation

Pre-operative Investigations

Nowadays it is unusual for anaesthetists to require 'routine' pre-operative investigations. History, examination and ward urine testing are a sufficient 'screen' in otherwise fit patients. Rather, investigations are used when there is a significant chance of uncovering an abnormality. Opinions vary as to what is 'significant' in this context, so the issuing of local guidelines often helps. An example of such guidelines is given in Table 6.5.

Table 6.5 Guidelines for the use of pre-operative investigations

Haemoglobin
  MANDATORY: History of or anticipated blood loss, e.g. menorrhagia or major surgery; 'cardiorespiratory disease'; female patients.
  UNNECESSARY: Healthy male patients and children having minor surgery.

Sickle test
  MANDATORY: Status not known in Afro-Caribbeans.
  UNNECESSARY: Status already known.

U&Es
  MANDATORY: Diuretic treatment, hypertension, heart or renal failure; major gut or urological surgery.
  UNNECESSARY: Most patients having minor procedures.

LFTs (including clotting screen)
  MANDATORY: Liver disease; unexplained fever after recent general anaesthetic; alcoholism, previous hepatitis.
  UNNECESSARY: As routine investigation.

Chest X-Ray
  MANDATORY: Heart failure, pulmonary disease with localizing signs.
  UNNECESSARY: Uncomplicated angina; asthma and COAD without localizing signs.

Neck X-Ray
  MANDATORY: Rheumatoid arthritis with unstable neck.
  UNNECESSARY: Rheumatoid arthritis with reduced neck movement.

Thoracic inlet X-ray
  MANDATORY: Thyroid enlargement.

ECG
  MANDATORY: Arrhythmias, angina, history of myocardial infarction, hypertension, heart failure.
  UNNECESSARY: Other patients and those in above categories with recent ECG.

Investigations may of course be done in other patients at the discretion of the clinician. The above guidelines are based on those issued to house surgeons at the Nottingham hospitals.

Special Situations

Day-case Surgery

Generally, patients are only considered for day-case surgery if they are otherwise completely fit or have a minor, well-controlled condition. In addition to the usual assessment, it is necessary to ascertain that the patient has undergone an appropriate period of starvation and has a responsible adult to act as an escort home and for overnight supervision. The patient must be advised not to drive or operate machinery for at least 24 hours.

Emergency Surgery

As always, the patient's general medical condition must be ascertained. In addition, especially in the case of abdominal emergencies or acute haemorrhage, a period of resuscitation may be required to restore circulating volume and/or extracellular fluid volume in general. Anaesthesia, whether general or regional, is hazardous in the hypovolaemic patient, so it is usual to complete rehydration and resuscitation before surgery takes place. It must be remembered that the majority of urgent cases, such as intestinal obstruction or perforated viscus, may be delayed for some hours while rehydration takes place; only occasionally, as in the case of a ruptured ectopic pregnancy or leaking aortic aneurysm, is speed important, and then resuscitation must proceed at the same time as anaesthesia and surgery.

The requirement for fluid replacement may be most easily gauged by the usual clinical approach; tachycardia, hypotension, cool peripheries and low urine output are all signs of a low circulating volume, while breathlessness, raised jugular venous pressure and crepitations in the lung fields indicate excessive fluid replacement. Investigations such as haematocrit, plasma urea and electrolytes, and chest X-ray may help, and the more complicated case may require pre-operative central venous pressure monitoring (see Chapter 5). Electrolyte concentrations may be deranged in these cases, and must be normalized before surgery.

Patients who present as emergencies are often in pain. Analgesia is as important before surgery as afterwards, remembering that hypovolaemic patients absorb intramuscular drugs slowly and unpredictably (see Chapter 7).

Fasting

Traditionally, patients having elective surgery in the morning have been starved of solids and liquids from midnight, and patients on the afternoon list have been thus starved from about 7 a.m. This is done, of course, to reduce the likelihood of regurgitation of stomach contents followed by aspiration of these contents into the lungs. There is now accumulating evidence that it is safe to anaesthetize patients within 3 hours of consumption of clear fluids, so several centres have adopted the practice of offering patients a drink at 6 a.m. (for the morning list) or mid-morning (for the afternoon list). Needless to say, this cup of tea is greatly appreciated by patients, and the break with years of entrenched hospital tradition has not proved difficult.

In the case of emergency surgery, the required period of starvation depends on the urgency of the proposed operation and the fact that pain, trauma and opioid analgesia all delay gastric emptying. If life, limb or vital organ function are threatened then the risk of aspiration becomes of secondary importance and surgery should proceed without delay. A rapid-sequence induction (see Chapter 1) is then obligatory.

Premedication

The principal purpose of premedication is to allay anxiety. Other drugs may be given at the same time for other purposes, and it is usually considered prudent for the patient to receive his usual drugs on the day of surgery (the obvious exception being oral hypoglycaemic agents).

Anxiolysis

Not all patients require an anxiolytic. Some patients are naturally calm, and the anaesthetist's visit (with appropriate explanation of what anaesthesia involves) often allays specific anxieties. Day-case patients do not normally receive anxiolytics as these delay recovery. Those who require an anxiolytic may be prescribed a benzodiazepine orally (temazepam and lorazepam are popular choices) or a potent opioid such as morphine intramuscularly; the latter may be given with or without hyoscine (which adds further sedation and also has anti-emetic properties).

Other Drugs Given with Premedication

An anti-emetic such as metoclopramide or prochlorperazine may be given. If the patient is at increased risk of aspiration of stomach contents (such as the pregnant patient or the patient with a hiatus hernia), then a histamine H_2 antagonist may help reduce stomach acidity. Transdermal glyceryl trinitrate patches are often prescribed for patients with coronary artery disease in the expectation that this will reduce myocardial ischaemia. Atropine is sometimes appropriate as a drying agent in upper respiratory tract endoscopies.

Children are a special case. Again, many require no sedation or anxiolysis, especially if appropriate explanation is given. Their natural fear of needles may be overcome by use of EMLA (eutectic mixture of local anaesthetics) cream – this cream is applied to the back of both hands and anaesthetizes the underlying skin. (This may also be used in adults with a particularly morbid fear of needles.) Small children often require atropine since they have strong vagal tone and are prone to bradycardia during anaesthesia. If sedation is required, the oral route is normally preferred, and trimeprazine (Vallergan) is popular.

Concluding Remarks

Pre-operative anaesthetic assessment and preparation require a thorough knowledge of the patient's general medical condition and its implications for anaesthesia and surgery. History, examination and appropriate use of investigations identify the vast majority of at-risk patients. Some of these patients will require adaptations to the anaesthetic technique or post-operative management while others will benefit from delaying surgery until their medical condition can be improved. The pre-operative visit also enables the anaesthetist to offer reassurance and prescribe premedication where appropriate.

Key Points

- In patients with co-existing medical conditions, consider not only the diagnosis but also the severity of the disease and the drugs being used to control it.

- The severity of the patient's general condition must always be balanced against the urgency and potential benefit of the surgery.

- When an operation is cancelled because of a patient's medical condition, consider how this condition may be improved before the patient is presented for surgery again.

- Try to use pre-operative investigations rationally.

- The anaesthetist's visit may allay anxiety at least as much as giving premedicant drugs.

Further Reading

Vickers, M.D., Jones, R.M. (eds) 1989: *Medicine for anaesthetists* (3rd edn). Oxford: Blackwell Science.

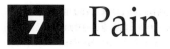 7 Pain

The Nature of Pain

Pain is a concept which can be difficult to define because of its subjective nature. Definitions tend to rely upon the response to a painful stimulus; thus, 'pain is a sensation which produces a reaction consisting of withdrawal response, metabolic response, hormonal response and conscious aversion'. Probably the simplest way to consider pain in the clinical context is as any stimulus perceived as unpleasant by the subject.

Pain and the Nervous System

Pain results from a noxious stimulus which causes tissue injury, resulting in the local release of chemicals such as bradykinin, substance P, histamine, prostaglandins and leukotrienes. These stimulate two distinct types of nerve fibres responsible for transmitting the sensation of pain to the central nervous system – the 'fast' Aδ fibres, responsible for sharp, acute, well-localized sensations and the 'slow' C fibres, which carry dull, poorly localized, visceral pain. These nerve impulses are then transmitted up the spinal cord to the higher centres or relayed via the anterior horn to provoke a reflex 'withdrawal' response.

Intervention at any point in this pathway will influence the severity of the pain. Thus aspirin, paracetamol and the non-steroidal anti-inflammatory drugs (NSAIDs) work by limiting the release of local, pain-producing chemicals, local anaesthesia blocks conduction of the pain impulse, and opioid drugs modulate spinal cord transmission and the perception of the stimulus in the higher centres. Some analgesic techniques, notably acupuncture and transcutaneous electrical nerve stimulation (TENS), probably work by stimulating nerve impulses which alter the sensitivity of the pathways in the spinal cord (the 'gate theory' of pain modulation).

Physiological Effects of Pain

Respiratory

Following major surgery, especially on the upper abdomen or chest, respiratory function is adversely affected for several days. Patients often complain that taking a deep breath makes their pain worse, and so tend to restrict themselves to shallow respiration. This inhibits re-expansion of areas of the lung which may have collapsed during anaesthesia, and prevents efficient gas exchange, leading to hypoxia. Obviously, if deep breathing causes pain then coughing is even worse, and patients are often understandably very reluctant to cough after major surgery, despite the best efforts of the physiotherapists! This results in the accumulation of bronchial secretions in the lungs, especially in smokers or those with chronic respiratory disease, increasing the likelihood of post-operative chest infections. There is good evidence to suggest that effective pain relief after surgery of this kind can reduce the risk of respiratory complications and shorten hospital stay.

Cardiovascular

The cardiovascular effects of pain are due to overactivity of the sympathetic nervous system, as pain causes secretion of catecholamines (adrenaline and noradrenaline) as part of the stress response (see below). The result is constriction of the peripheral blood vessels, tachycardia and hypertension. Although well tolerated by healthy individuals, this combination causes a considerable increase in the work done by the heart, and this may cause problems in patients with pre-existing heart disease, especially myocardial ischaemia. It is well recognized that patients with established ischaemic heart disease are at considerably higher risk from peri-operative myocardial infarction in the first few days following surgery.

Hormonal

The stress response to surgery is a well-documented combination of metabolic and endocrine changes which can be characterized by a rise in catabolic hormones (cortisol, catecholamines and glucagon) and a fall in anabolic hormones (insulin and testosterone). The overall effect is to mobilize energy substrates from storage and make them available to healing tissue. It seems, therefore, that this stress response may be a useful reaction to the trauma of surgery; it may be an over-reaction, however, as there is plenty of evidence to suggest that it can be 'damped down' without adversely affecting healing, and with the benefits that accrue from minimizing abnormal hormonal changes. Diabetic patients, particularly, can have their blood sugar control thrown into disarray by the hyperglycaemic outcome of the stress response. Intra- and post-operative analgesia, especially when provided by regional or local anaesthetic techniques, has been shown to reduce the stress response to manageable levels, so benefiting this kind of patient.

Psychological Effects of Pain

Of course, even if pain produced no unwanted physiological effects, its very nature makes it something that, as caring physicians, we should work hard to abolish. Not surprisingly, most people who have a painful experience try hard to avoid putting themselves in the same position again. Patients who experience severe pain as a result of investigation or treatment are far less likely to seek medical help in the future and, at its worst, this sort of reaction can develop into a pathological fear of hospitals or doctors. Pain has a powerful effect on the mind; for many people, their earliest memory is of the fear and pain associated with a childhood operation or hospital visit.

It is surprising that, even in this enlightened age, pain is often afforded a low priority when hospital staff are treating patients. The belief that post-operative pain is inevitable, or even that pain is somehow good for you, still lingers in some quarters. Only 150 years ago, the introduction of pain relief for labouring mothers was strongly opposed by the Church, and military leaders felt that soldiers receiving anaesthesia for field surgery would become soft and lose their fighting spirit. If you think that this kind of attitude is now defunct, it is worth remembering that, until a few years ago, it was common practice not to give analgesia when operating on neonates as it was felt that they would not 'remember' their pain, and that there is still some debate as to whether babies in intensive care units need pain relief during invasive procedures. Many surgical wards still use archaic methods of analgesia, and these do not usually change until the consultant surgeon goes through agonies after his cholecystectomy!

Measuring Pain

It should be self-evident that, if we are to make progress in treating or preventing pain, we must be able to measure it. After all, we would not get far in the management of diabetes if we were unable to measure serum glucose levels accurately. Unfortunately, the measurement of pain is a notoriously difficult task as pain is, by definition, a subjective experience. One thing is for sure; attempts to measure a patient's pain by another person, however well trained, tend to lead to underestimation. The best person to assess pain (or the effects of pain relief) is the patient himself, and a large majority of clinicians and researchers use the patient's own estimate to tell them how well they are succeeding in their attempts to provide analgesia.

Patient scoring systems vary; for ease of use, some centres use a method whereby the patient scores his pain on a discrete point count (0 = no pain, 1 = mild discomfort . . . . . ranging up to 5 = severe pain). The most commonly used system, however, is the 10 cm linear analogue pain score. The patient is asked to make a mark on a line, one extreme of which represents no pain,

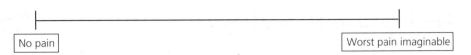

Figure 7.1 Ten-centimetre analogue pain scale.

and the other the worst pain the patient can imagine (Figure 7.1). The distance along the line can then be measured, and the degree of pain translated into a numerical value.

Acute Pain

Acute Pain and the Anaesthetist

The anaesthetist spends a considerable amount of time trying to prevent or treat acute pain, and generally finds it in three locations: the post-operative recovery unit, the accident and emergency department and the labour suite. In this section we will first look at some of the features which differentiate these types of pain, and then examine ways of dealing with them.

Post-operative Pain

The most common pain met by the anaesthetist, post-operative pain, is best dealt with by preventing it happening in the first place (see 'pre-emptive analgesia'). The patient who wakes up in severe pain following surgery can be a difficult problem, and the mainstay of dealing with this sort of occurrence is the intravenous administration of opioid drugs such as morphine, large doses of which may be necessary. Certainly, if a patient is discharged from the recovery unit in pain, then the chances of analgesia becoming effective on the ward, where nurse:patient ratios are lower, nurse training in pain relief is often poor and intravenous access may not be available, are negligible.

Trauma Pain

Anaesthetists may be called down to the accident and emergency department specifically to help with a pain problem, but are more likely to encounter a trauma patient in pain when in the process of resuscitation or preparation for theatre. It is important that analgesia in these circumstances does not interfere with the resuscitation process or mask important diagnostic signs in the patient. For example, the use of intravenous morphine to treat a man with a fractured femur, shock and head injury may lower his blood pressure further, depress his level of consciousness, interfere with neurological observations and increase the risk of regurgitation and aspiration of gastric contents. It is still important to treat pain in these circumstances, however, and a nerve block with local anaesthetics (see below) is often the technique of choice.

Labour Pain

The pain of childbirth is, at its worst, one of the most severe pains that can be experienced, and very few mothers are lucky enough to go through labour without the need for some form of analgesia. Several features distinguish the pain of labour from the other forms of pain: it gets worse, not better, with time; it is non-pathological, and associated with a happy outcome; its relief must not result in compromise to the baby, and should not interfere with the ability of the mother to share in the birth experience. This means that the ideal pain relief in labour must be very potent, very safe and not have any depressant effect upon the central nervous system. This is where regional block, in the form of epidural or spinal anaesthesia, comes into its own, and this is discussed further in the chapter on local anaesthesia.

Drugs

Detailed pharmacology of the important analgesic drugs is dealt with elsewhere in this book (see Chapter 3). Here we outline the roles that different drugs have to play in the management of acute pain, whether singly or in combination.

Simple Analgesia

Simple analgesic drugs such as aspirin and paracetamol are of little use when dealing with severe pain. They are not strong enough and they can usually only be administered orally, a route which is certainly not practicable following major surgery. However, it is important not to forget these drugs later in the post-operative period; while recovering from painful surgery, most patients need a 'halfway' drug to tide them over the period between opioid usage and total freedom from pain. As well as paracetamol and aspirin, there is a wide range of medications which combine one of these agents with such drugs as codeine or dextropropoxyphene, and these combinations are often clinically beneficial.

Non-steroidal Anti-inflammatory Drugs (NSAIDs)

This wide-ranging group of drugs, used for many years to treat arthritis and other musculoskeletal disorders, is now finding a role, often in combination with opioids, in the management of post-operative pain. Recent additions to the range, such as diclofenac and ketorolac, have more powerful analgesic properties than their ancestors, and have the added advantage that they can be administered via a variety of routes including intramuscular, intravenous and rectal. Other preparations can be applied topically.

NSAIDs have well recognized side-effects, the most notorious being gastric irritation and haemorrhage. They also interfere with platelet function and may exacerbate asthma and renal failure.

Opioids

Morphine and its derivatives have been used since the days of the ancient Greeks to relieve pain and remain the standard against which other analgesic techniques are measured. When used in the correct dose by the appropriate route, opioids are safe and very effective, but in practice their performance is often disappointing. The reasons for this are mostly organizational, and are discussed below. The detailed pharmacology of the opioids is dealt with in Chapter 3.

Of the drugs available, morphine is the most commonly prescribed in the UK, and has a duration of action of about 3–4 hours following a single intramuscular dose. Papaveretum is a drug containing the hydrochlorides of the alkaloids of opium, standardized so that its anhydrous morphine content is 50 per cent; it has declined in popularity since one of its components, noscapine, was implicated in causing germ cell abnormalities, but it is now available in a noscapine-free preparation. Diamorphine (heroin) is a powerful analgesic with some advantages over morphine; its association with addiction and abuse have, probably unfairly, somewhat restricted its use. Pethidine, used especially in labour, is slightly shorter-acting and has atropine-like properties, causing bronchodilation, tachycardia and reduction in secretions. Pethidine derivatives, such as fentanyl and alfentanil, are very potent, short-acting opioids that tend to be used intraoperatively, although they can be used post-operatively via the epidural or spinal routes (see below).

Opioid drugs may be administered via a variety of routes.

PARENTERAL

The 'standard' post-operative opioid regimen consists of instructions to the nursing staff to give a fixed dose of morphine by intramuscular injection when requested by the patient, with a minimum interval between doses. This type of regimen has many drawbacks (see below). The intramuscular route is painful and invasive and, when given this way, morphine has a lag time of some 20 minutes before starting to work. More importantly, for a drug to be taken up into the bloodstream from muscle, it is essential that the muscle is well perfused, and this is not the case when tissue perfusion is poor, as may occur after trauma, blood loss or prolonged surgery. The intravenous route has many benefits: the drug may be given painlessly through an indwelling cannula; the dose can be titrated against the rapid response to give the desired effect; and there is no reliance on adequate tissue perfusion.

The fact that, at the time of writing, most opioids are given on the ward by painful injection into the muscle owes far more to the persistence of archaic practice than to any scientific approach to pain relief. With the advent of better organization of post-operative care, the intramuscular route will probably go the way of the ether bottle in modern anaesthetic practice.

INFUSIONS

The increasing use of the intravenous route has led to wider adoption of continuous infusion techniques for giving opioids. These have the obvious advantage that they are designed to maintain a constant blood level of analgesia, rather than the wildly fluctuating levels achieved with bolus injection. Unfortunately, individuals vary considerably in their response to a given level of opioid; the dose that relieves pain in patient A will leave patient B in agony and put patient C into severe respiratory depression. Contrary to popular belief, body weight is actually a very poor predictor of requirements for opioids.

PATIENT-CONTROLLED ANALGESIA (PCA) (FIGURE 7.2)

PCA is a technique that was designed to overcome the limitations described above. The idea works like this: only the patient knows how much pain he

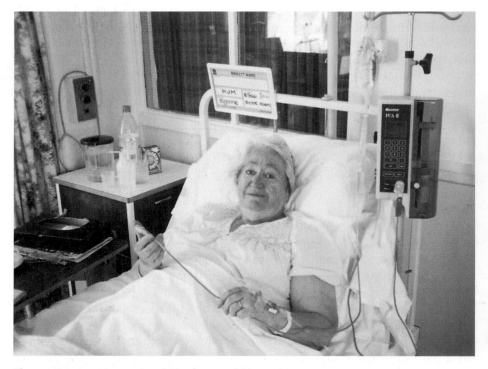

Figure 7.2 A patient using PCA after total hip replacement.

Table 7.1 Opioid doses for adults

	Intramuscular use	PCA use (all with a 5 min lock-out time)
Morphine	10–15 mg 3 hourly	1 mg
Papaveretum	15–20 mg 3 hourly	2 mg
Diamorphine	5–10 mg 2 hourly	0.5 mg
Pethidine	75–150 mg 2 hourly	10 mg

is suffering, and only the patient can determine how effective a dose of morphine has been in relieving that pain. Therefore, give the patient the means to treat his own pain. In practice, this is achieved by filling a syringe with a large quantity of morphine and connecting it to an intravenous cannula. The patient is given a button which, when pressed, delivers a fixed, small dose of morphine. The machine 'locks out' for a short period of time to give the dose a chance to achieve its effect (usually five minutes), and then the patient may take another dose if needed. A typical prescription would allow 1 mg of morphine to be taken every five minutes, thus allowing a patient as much as 12 mg/h. A patient with PCA left to his own devices will take large doses of morphine in the first few hours after surgery, gradually tailing down as the pain naturally abates until he is pressing the button only once or twice per hour. Patients using PCA often have higher pain scores than those receiving other forms of analgesic treatment, but express much greater satisfaction. This is believed to be for two reasons; the patient is more confident because he has control over his analgesic therapy, and is also able to titrate the dose to achieve satisfactory analgesia with the minimum of side-effects (particularly nausea).

Adult doses of the more common opioids are listed in Table 7.1.

EPIDURAL/SPINAL

Receptors for opioids are found in high concentrations in the spinal cord, and small doses of these drugs can have profound analgesic effects when administered into the epidural or intrathecal (spinal) regions. A dose of morphine as small as 0.2 mg (one-fiftieth of the intramuscular dose) can produce highly effective pain relief for 24 hours following lower abdominal surgery. No advance is without its price, however, and sudden onset of respiratory depression has been reported with these techniques, often some hours after administration. This problem occurs particularly in elderly patients or those who have had concomitant sedative drugs or opioids by other routes. Opinion is divided as to whether patients treated in this way need high-dependency care or can be nursed on a general ward.

Side-effects of Opioids

The adverse effects of opioids are listed in Table 7.2. Of particular relevance to their clinical use are the risks of nausea and respiratory depression.

Table 7.2 Adverse effects of opioid drugs

Sedation
Respiratory depression
Nausea and vomiting
Dysphoria
Itching
Urinary retention
Histamine release
Miosis

NAUSEA AND VOMITING

All opioids in use at present can cause these most unpleasant side-effects, although constant efforts are being made to split the emetic and analgesic properties of these drugs. Nausea and vomiting can be so distressing to patients that they will forgo pain relief rather than suffer the consequences.

Patients who have a history of vomiting after opioids should be pretreated with an anti-emetic such as prochlorperazine, cyclizine or metoclopramide. These drugs may also be effective if used to treat vomiting once it has occurred, but really refractory cases may need a more powerful agent such as ondansetron.

RESPIRATORY DEPRESSION

The most feared of opioid-induced adverse effects, there is no doubt that severe respiratory depression has caused, and will continue to cause, death in frail patients in the first few days after surgery. Respiratory depression goes hand-in-hand with sedation and is dose-dependent although, as implied earlier, the dose that may produce this effect differs markedly between individuals. It is important to bear in mind that not only respiratory rate, but also depth, may be affected, and a patient may have a significant reduction in minute volume with a near-normal respiratory rate. Except when spinal opioids are used, respiratory depression does not happen suddenly, and its gradual onset can be detected as long as the patient is adequately monitored – it is therefore essential that all patients receiving opioid drugs are carefully and frequently monitored for signs of excessive sedation and respiratory inadequacy.

OPIOID ANTAGONISTS

If marked sedation or respiratory depression is seen in a patient who has had opioids, the most effective and rapid treatment is to give an intravenous bolus of naloxone, a specific opioid antagonist. The results are dramatic, with a previously unrousable patient suddenly sitting up and opening his eyes within one minute of treatment. Two important points should be borne in mind when using naloxone, however. First, naloxone also reverses the analgesic effects of the opioid, so a patient's pain may return and be difficult to treat: second, the half-life of naloxone is quite short – this may result in a patient slipping back into a comatose state 15–30 minutes after a dose of naloxone has appeared to work. The patient who has been treated with naloxone therefore needs close observation, and further doses should be on hand. The normal dose is 0.1 mg iv, repeated until the desired effect is achieved.

Local Anaesthesia

The use of local anaesthetic drugs is dealt with in detail in Chapter 2. In general, the judicious use of local anaesthetics during a surgical procedure can transform the immediate post-operative period. Techniques ranging from epidural block to simple wound infiltration have proved very effective, and are limited only by the relatively short duration of action of current drugs, which usually wear off within 2–6 hours. Leaving a catheter *in situ*, as with epidural analgesia, gets around this problem by allowing for 'top-ups' of local anaesthetic to be given at regular intervals.

Drug Combinations

There is no doubt that analgesia is best achieved by attacking the pain pathway at several different points along its length. For example, a patient undergoing major abdominal surgery may be given a bolus of intravenous morphine in theatre, and an epidural catheter inserted before surgery to provide an intra-operative conduction block. A non-steroidal anti-inflammatory drug such a diclofenac may be given during the procedure with regular repeat doses written up, and the patient started on PCA with morphine before return to the ward. This rather poly-pharmaceutical approach means that smaller doses of the individual drugs can be used, so limiting adverse effects, while better analgesia can be achieved than with any individual drug alone.

Pre-emptive Analgesia

Pain is far easier to prevent than to treat, and all anaesthetists strive to wake a patient up in as comfortable a condition as possible. Opioid drugs are used intraoperatively as an important part of the anaesthetic technique, the powerful, short-acting agents such as fentanyl being particularly useful for this purpose.

Organizational Factors

Recovery Units

The role of the recovery unit is discussed in Chapter 1. One of the most important roles of the recovery nurse is to ensure that patients leaving the

POST-OPERATIVE PAIN ASSESSMENT CHART

GUIDE TO NURSING OBSERVATIONS

PATIENT STICKER

All observations: $\frac{1}{2}$ hrly for 2 h, hrly for 4 h, 2 hrly thereafter

If treatment required: return to frequent observations, at least hrly, until problem rectified

RESPIRATORY RATE

While the patient is at rest count rate for one full minute

SEDATION SCORE (enter as **O** in boxes 0–3)

AWAKE	0
DROWSY	1
SLEEPING / EASILY ROUSED	2
SLEEPING / DIFFICULT TO ROUSE	3

PAIN SCORE (enter as **X** in boxes 0–3)
After getting patient to take a deep breath, cough or move, ask: *'Which of these best describes how you feel?'*

NO PAIN	0
MILD PAIN	1
MODERATE PAIN	2
SEVERE PAIN	3

If any score is 2 or 3 take appropriate action and recommence hourly observations

Date																								
Time																								
3																								
2																								
1																								
0																								
Nausea Score																								
Vol in Syringe																								
Rate																								
PCA tries/good																								
Action taken																								

CONTACT PERSONNEL

During working hours: Prescribing anaesthetist or acute pain nurse (bleep)
After hours or urgent: Duty anaesthetist (bleep)

Figure 7.3 A pain-scoring chart for use on the post-operative ward.

unit are as comfortable as possible, and to this end many units allow staff to give intravenous boluses of opioid drugs, this being the quickest and most effective way to achieve analgesia in a patient who wakes up in pain.

Acute Pain Team

Recognizing that post-operative wards are poorly equipped, and the staff often poorly motivated to deal with pain, many hospitals are establishing acute pain teams. Usually under the control of a consultant anaesthetist, and run by anaesthetists, surgeons and nurses, the acute pain team fulfils a consultative role, visiting wards routinely or at the request of nursing staff to assess analgesia, adjust infusions or PCA machines and suggest other treatments for patients with continuing pain. The other main function of such a team is educational, running teach-ins on modern analgesic techniques and encouraging improvements in monitoring pain, such as the introduction of pain charts on which levels of pain, sedation and nausea may be scored regularly (Figure 7.3).

High-dependency Units

Some modern analgesic methods, such as the combined use of epidural local anaesthetic and opioid drugs, require more careful supervision than can be achieved on a general ward. These patients are best nursed in an environment with continuous monitoring and a high nurse:patient ratio. These high-dependency units (HDUs) are becoming increasingly common, and provide both a 'halfway house' for the patient transferring from a recovery unit to a general ward, and a useful training facility for nurses and junior doctors learning to manage the immediate complications of major surgery.

Chronic Pain

In recent years, anaesthetists have become more involved in the management of chronic pain. This has led to participation in activities traditionally shunned by anaesthetists: GP referrals, outpatient clinics and waiting lists. The successful treatment of patients with long-standing debilitating pain is, however, one of the most satisfying features of modern anaesthetic practice, and the gradual appreciation that a large number of such patients exist has led to considerable expansion in the number and size of pain clinics across the UK.

Pain clinics are usually multidisciplinary and often include the services of nurses, physiotherapists, pharmacists, and psychologists. Access to radiological and surgical services is essential. Drugs, although important, are not the mainstay of chronic pain treatment, and patients often require nerve blocks, transcutaneous nerve stimulation (TENS), acupuncture or behavioural therapy.

The Patients

A wide variety of patients can find their way into the care of the chronic pain specialist, but they can be broadly categorized as follows:

Musculoskeletal disorders are probably the most common problems encountered, and these tend to be concentrated in the lower thoracolumbar spine. Backache is very common, notoriously difficult to treat, and can be quite debilitating. By the time the sufferer reaches the pain clinic most standard treatments have been tried, and epidural injections of steroids with local anaesthetic drugs are often the next step. Physiotherapists are often involved in the care of these patients, and other support staff such as dietitians and chiropractors may also have a role.

Persistent post-operative wound pain is often due to entrapment of a nerve or neuroma formation. These often respond to local injections of steroids or specific nerve blocks, but sometimes require surgical re-exploration.

Central pain states are a group of disorders in which pain probably arises centrally, rather than from a peripheral stimulus. They include post-herpetic neuralgia and phantom limb pain and can be very refractory to treatment. Anticonvulsant drugs such as phenytoin and carbamazepine can be effective and, along with many other chronic pain conditions, tricyclic antidepressants may have a useful part to play.

Cancer pain is a distressing symptom which often blights the short life-span of patients with terminal disease. Due to bony infiltration, local tissue destruction or involvement of major nerves such as the splanchnic, terminal pain often needs to be treated with very high doses of opioid drugs, given either systemically or epidurally. Obliteration of affected nerves with alcohol, phenol or electric current may be effective.

Key Points

- Pain is subjective – only the patient can appreciate the degree of his/her pain.
- Pain has adverse physiological and psychological effects.
- It is easier to prevent pain than to treat it once it is established.
- 'Traditional' post-operative analgesic regimens often provide poor pain relief.
- Opioid drugs remain the mainstay of treatment of acute pain. Modern methods of administration including PCA and epidural/spinal use have greatly improved their clinical efficacy.
- Opioid side effects are predictable and dose-related.
- Combinations of opioids and other analgesic methods can be particularly effective.
- Organizational factors are important when treating post-operative pain. Acute pain teams are becoming more common.
- Chronic pain is often multifactorial, and can be very difficult to treat.

Further Reading

Cousins, M.J., Bridenbaugh, P.L. 1988: *Neural blockade in clinical anaesthesia and management of pain* (2nd edn). Philadelphia: Lippincott.

Hosking, J., Welchew, E. 1985: *Postoperative pain*. London: Faber and Faber.

Wall, P.D., Melzack, R. 1994: *Textbook of pain* (3rd edn). Edinburgh: Churchill Livingstone.

8 The Post-operative Period

Introduction

It was not very long ago that the anaesthetist's responsibility ended when the patient was lifted off the operating table. There were no recovery rooms in British hospitals until the early 1950s, and it was not until a government building regulation of 1967 that there was official recognition of the necessity to have a properly equipped and staffed recovery area. The practice of sending a patient straight back to the ward within minutes of the end of an operation therefore persisted until quite recently, and overcoming this custom required a recognition not only that certain post-operative complications occurred but also that they might be prevented or treated by close observation in the first hour or so after the operation.

This chapter is therefore largely concerned with the complications associated with anaesthesia. Complications do not, of course, occur only in the recovery room and the anaesthetist should also take an interest in what happens to the patient after return to the ward, since his activities can influence the patient's recovery over several days. The patient who requires intensive care post-operatively is dealt with in Chapter 9.

It is hard to establish the exact incidence of complications because it is often difficult to define exactly when, for example, a minor degree of hypoxia becomes a 'complication'. It is safe to assume that at least 20 per cent of patients have a complication, of which the majority relate to the respiratory or cardiovascular systems. About 1 in 2000 patients suffer cardiac arrest in the recovery room, and about 1 in 6000 die there. Most complications occur in patients who already have major disease in the respiratory or cardiovascular systems.

In the following sections, post-operative complications are categorized by body system, to aid discussion.

The Respiratory System

Hypoxia

Hypoxia is a common occurrence in the early post-operative period. It has recently been recognized more frequently because of the increased use of the

Table 8.1 Some causes of hypoxia in the post-operative period (see text for details)

Reduced central drive to ventilation	—	drugs
	—	CO_2 washout
Residual effect of muscle relaxant		
Upper airway obstruction		
Bronchospasm		
Increased ventilation–perfusion mismatch		
Reduced functional residual capacity		
Diffusion hypoxia		
Aspiration of blood/stomach contents		
Pneumothorax		
Pain		
Sputum retention		
Pulmonary embolus		

pulse oximeter – as discussed in Chapter 5, this device is far more sensitive than 'naked-eye' recognition of clinical cyanosis. A list of causes of post-operative hypoxia is given in Table 8.1.

Impaired function of the respiratory centre in the brain occurs with appropriate therapeutic amounts of opioids, barbiturates, and volatile anaesthetics. This may cause problems in patients with reduced respiratory reserve or with unusual sensitivity to these drugs. Reduction in respiratory minute volume may also occur following enforced hyperventilation imposed by the anaesthetist.

The patient may still be partly paralysed by a muscle relaxant on arrival in the recovery area. This should not occur if an anticholinesterase has been given and a peripheral nerve stimulator has been used properly (see Chapter 5), but remains an occasional clinical problem. Upper airway obstruction may occur for a variety of reasons, the common ones being laryngeal spasm, occlusion of the pharynx by reduced muscle tone, and material such as blood.

Inhalation of blood (following, for example, tonsillectomy) or stomach contents (following regurgitation) remains an important cause of 'anaesthetic' mortality, accounting for some 20–25 per cent of such deaths.

Various physiological changes occur in the lungs following anaesthesia and surgery. Perhaps most important is a fall in functional residual capacity, which may be reduced by up to 30 per cent after abdominal surgery. This, together with other changes, such as impaired pulmonary hypoxic vasoconstriction, contributes to the increase in ventilation–perfusion mismatch which is a cause of post-operative hypoxia.

Diffusion hypoxia may occur for 5–10 minutes following the discontinuation of nitrous oxide. This phenomenon is discussed in Chapter 3.

Acute pathology of the lungs may occur in the early post-operative period. Bronchospasm may follow the injection of drugs which release histamine or instrumentation of the airway (including tracheal intubation), and pneumothorax may follow positive pressure ventilation, especially if high inflation pressures have been used or there is pre-existing pathology such as an emphysematous bulla. These conditions are managed in the same way as when they present on the medical ward.

Pain, if inadequately controlled, may contribute to hypoxia. Following abdominal surgery, pain may prevent full expansion of the lungs and predispose to sputum retention, airways collapse and pneumonia.

Fortunately, the wise anaesthetist does not have to agonize over each of these problems with each individual patient. Simple manoeuvres help considerably, whatever the cause of the hypoxia. Increasing the inspired concentration of oxygen helps in virtually any situation, although care should be taken with the *rare* patient who is dependent on hypoxic drive to maintain ventilation. It will be obvious that many of the problems discussed above continue for some time after the patient has left the recovery room, and it is becoming increasingly common for anaesthetists to prescribe oxygen for several days in high-risk patients. The co-operation of both patient and nurses is improved by prescribing oxygen at night, as this is when the majority of documented episodes of hypoxia occur.

Allowing the patient to recover in the lateral position not only reduces the probability that material will be inhaled, but also helps to keep the pharyngeal lumen open and reduces the work of breathing (particularly in the obese patient).

Does any of this matter? Do minor degrees of hypoxia have an adverse effect on the average patient? Common sense suggests that it does matter, and for once the findings of clinical research agree with common sense! Episodes of post-operative hypoxia have been documented to correspond with episodes of myocardial ischaemia, and myocardial ischaemia is known to predispose to low cardiac output (impairing healing of wounds and anastomoses) and myocardial infarction. Generations of house surgeons have felt victimized because patients always seem to develop haemodynamic problems in the middle of the night, and we now know that this impression is accurate, since the majority of episodes of hypoxia occur at night.

Hypercapnia

Oxygen delivery is, of course, only one aspect of respiratory function, and carbon dioxide elimination must also be considered. The partial pressure of carbon dioxide (CO_2) increases whenever the minute volume of ventilation falls. Thus, it occurs particularly when drugs have been given which depress respiratory drive. This occurs to some degree with virtually any anaesthetic agent, and particularly when opioids are given. Carbon dioxide retention may occur also when a patient with chronic bronchitis who is dependent on hypoxic drive is given an excessive concentration of oxygen to breathe. This is particularly likely to happen when these patients are allowed to breathe from a 'variable-performance' oxygen mask such as the MC mask rather than a 'fixed-performance' device such as the Ventimask, which delivers a concentration of oxygen which does not vary with the patient's inspiratory flow. However, *most* bronchitic patients do not rely on hypoxic drive, and do not need a restricted

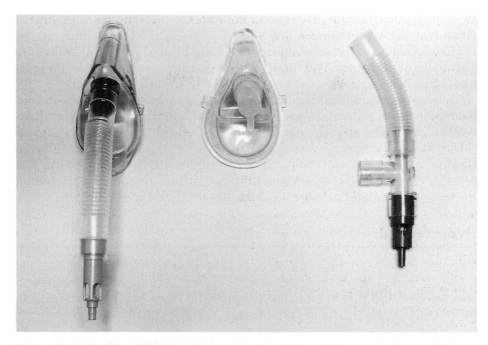

Figure 8.1 Examples of fixed-performance and variable-performance oxygen masks. (From left) Ventimask (fixed), MC mask (variable) and 'T-piece' systems used with LMA or tracheal tube (variable).

inspired oxygen concentration. Examples of variable-performance and fixed-performance oxygen delivery devices are shown in Figure 8.1.

The consequences of CO_2 retention include effects on the cardiovascular system (hypertension, tachycardia, arrhythmias) as well as the effects of CO_2 narcosis. This narcosis is a cause of delayed recovery of consciousness and puts the patient at risk by delaying recovery of protective reflexes. It is an apparent paradox that this problem may be increasing with the increased use of pulse oximeters (see Chapter 5). A normal oxygen saturation, as demonstrated by the pulse oximeter, may deceive the unwise observer into thinking that respiratory function is normal, when there may be considerable CO_2 retention. The only way to confirm normal respiratory function is by measuring arterial blood gases.

The Cardiovascular System

Hypotension

The most common cause of post-operative hypotension is a low blood volume. This may be because of blood loss, often occult, or loss of other fluids, for example if significant mesenteric oedema occurs after abdominal surgery. It is not uncommon for insidious bleeding to be missed because the hypotension is wrongly attributed to the residual effects of the anaesthetic. Post-operative hypotension is due to hypovolaemia until proved otherwise.

That said, the hypotensive effects of anaesthetic drugs may linger into the post-operative period. This applies particularly to epidural and spinal techniques.

Sometimes a cardiac cause for the hypotension needs to be considered. Examples are an arrhythmia (such as fast atrial fibrillation or complete heart block), myocardial ischaemia, or possibly infarction.

Most causes of hypotension respond well to a head-down tilt and administration of intravenous fluids (although care should be taken if a cardiac cause is suspected). Oxygen should always be given because hypotension increases ventilation–perfusion mismatching.

Hypertension

Probably the most common cause of hypertension in this group of patients is pain, and on recovering consciousness the patient may become hypertensive before being able to articulate his problem. Pain, of course, is treatable by giving analgesics. The problem is that hypertension may also be caused by hypoxia or hypercapnia, both of which are accentuated by opioid treatment. The decision of whether or not to give opioids to a semi-conscious patient in the recovery room is often difficult.

Sometimes, other causes of hypertension need to be considered. A full bladder may cause blood pressure to rise, and is easily managed by passing a urinary catheter or releasing the clamp on a catheter which is already in place. Very rare causes include metabolic derangements such as malignant hyperpyrexia or thyrotoxic crisis.

Arrhythmias

Cardiac arrhythmias are most likely to occur when there is pre-existing cardiac disease. Precipitating factors include acute myocardial ischaemia, perhaps provoked by pain, and disturbances such as hypoxia, hypercapnia or electrolyte abnormality. Drugs may be responsible, for example if adrenaline has been infiltrated during surgery or if halothane has been used (see Chapter 3). Some operations are more likely than others to be associated with arrhythmias, and these include dental and thoracic surgery.

Major Cardiac Events

This phrase has been coined to cover events such as myocardial infarction, unstable angina, pulmonary oedema and ventricular tachycardia occurring in the post-operative period. Considerable effort has gone into attempting to predict which patients are particularly at risk from these complications, with the assumption that by paying special attention to the at-risk group the incidence will be reduced.

The first risk factors to be identified were the pre-operative factors. The exact details vary from one group of researchers to another, but all are agreed on two factors: recent myocardial infarction and significant heart failure. 'Significant' heart failure in this context means pulmonary oedema, gallop rhythm or raised jugular venous pressure. It is obvious that a patient's prognosis will be improved by treating heart failure and delaying elective surgery after recent myocardial infarction.

Intraoperative risk factors involve mainly abnormalities of haemodynamics. Tachycardia, hypotension and hypertension should be avoided.

Post-operative risk factors are attracting attention at the moment. Prolonged post-operative ischaemia or tachycardia predispose to infarction in the first few post-operative days, and it is logical to expect high-risk patients to have access to high-dependency units where they can be observed closely for early signs of hypoxia, myocardial ischaemia, etc., and appropriate treatment instituted promptly.

Pulmonary Embolism

Death from pulmonary embolism, which occurs typically when the patient is well on the way to recovery after surgery, can be particularly distressing for both family and hospital staff. The impact of anaesthetic technique on its incidence is not major, but the anaesthetist can do his best to ensure adequate hydration and early ambulation. Some workers believe that regional anaesthetic techniques reduce the incidence of deep venous thrombosis when compared with general anaesthesia.

'Minor' Vascular Complications

Phlebitis and haematomas may follow venepuncture and intravenous infusions. Some instances of phlebitis persist for several weeks or months, and sympathy and analgesia are all that can be offered. Further complications may arise when an arterial line has been used. There is a significant incidence of occlusion of the artery, but these are rarely clinically important. Occasionally, injections are given erroneously into an arterial line and this may be followed by significant spasm, thrombosis and ischaemia in the limb. The arterial line should be labelled clearly so that all staff looking after the patient are aware of its nature.

The Gastro-intestinal System

Nausea and Vomiting

This is a particularly distressing complication for the patient. The patient who says 'Doctor, I was terribly unwell after my last anaesthetic' doesn't mean that she spent several days on intensive care and was at death's door. No, she means she vomited a lot, and to her this is very important.

Some patients are more likely than others to be sick after anaesthetics. Females more than males, the young more than the old, the obese, those who suffer from motion sickness – all these are likely to suffer from post-operative nausea. Some operations are likely to provoke this complication; these include operations on the eye, middle ear, pelvic organs and biliary tree. The exact anaesthetic technique used probably does not affect the incidence of nausea and vomiting very much, especially since opioids are the most potent cause of vomiting and it is difficult to avoid the use of opioids during surgery.

The treatment of post-operative nausea and vomiting is discussed in Chapter 3.

Passive Regurgitation

Although nausea and vomiting are dreaded by the patient, it is passive regurgitation which is more sinister from the anaesthetist's viewpoint. Stomach contents in the pharynx may be inhaled into the lungs when protective reflexes such as the gag reflex and the cough reflex are inhibited by anaesthesia. Inhalation of stomach contents may in turn lead to severe, life-threatening chemical pneumonia.

Factors predisposing to passive regurgitation are dealt with in Chapter 1. The risk of passive regurgitation may be reduced by awareness of the hazard, by taking precautions such as tracheal intubation with a rapid-sequence induction (see Chapter 1), and by allowing the at-risk patient to recover in the lateral position.

Liver Failure

The issue of halothane hepatitis is discussed in Chapter 4. It may interest the reader to know that the major culprit for liver damage amongst the inhalational agents is chloroform, which nowadays is used only in novels. It is impressive that protagonists in crime novels always achieve a smooth induction with chloroform and also avoid the long-term complications such as liver failure.

The Genito-urinary System

Oliguria

The causes of oliguria are well known to most clinical medical students. Pre-renal causes (hypovolaemia) are common in the post-operative period, because of unpredictable degrees of post-operative blood loss, oedema formation, and insensible water loss. Renal causes include mismatched blood transfusion, and bile salt precipitation in the renal tubules in the patient with obstructive jaundice. Post-renal causes include prostatism and of course that old favourite, the blocked or misplaced catheter. It seems to be a necessary part of each houseman's career to miss the catheter which has fallen out of the bladder until the patient's bladder has filled up to the level of the umbilicus.

Prevention of oliguria involves, most importantly, ensuring adequate hydration, and this is a convenient point to discuss the issue of *post-operative fluid balance*. Patients who have had major surgery, particularly inside the abdomen, require intravenous fluids for a few days afterwards. The usual requirements are 2–3 litres per day, but this may be increased if there are abnormal losses from drains, fistulae, etc. Crystalloid is normally appropriate unless there is bleeding. A judicious combination of normal saline, 5 per cent dextrose and/or dextrose saline may be chosen, with the precise detail dictated by frequent estimation of plasma electrolyte concentration. A typical 'recipe' would comprise one litre of normal saline and two litres of 5 per cent dextrose for the 24-hour period. Five per cent dextrose provides water because the dextrose is metabolized rapidly, and the saline provides the appropriate amount of sodium to replace that lost in urine, oedema fluid, etc. If 5 per cent dextrose alone is used, the patient becomes hyponatraemic and develops cerebral oedema as the water passes into the intracellular space.

The addition of potassium to the maintenance fluids is normally not necessary for the first 24–48 hours. Although the post-operative period is characterized by potassium loss in the urine, it appears that enough potassium is mobilized from the intracellular space to maintain normal plasma concentration for a day or so. Again, guidance will be obtained from plasma electrolyte estimation but normally 20–40 mmol are required in 24 hours when potassium replacement becomes necessary.

The adequacy of fluid replacement may be gauged clinically (see Chapter 6), and by reference to the fluid balance chart which is usually found hanging on the end of the patient's bed. This assures the anxious house officer that the fluid input is maintaining adequate urine output (about 30 mL/h). In difficult cases, monitoring of central venous pressure will help, and a CVP line will often have been placed by the anaesthetist. Diuretics may be used judiciously in the elderly or unfit patient.

Problems with the Reproductive System

Giving an anaesthetic to a patient in the first trimester of pregnancy increases the risk of spontaneous abortion, and in the later stages of pregnancy increases the risk of premature labour. Anaesthesia in the pregnant patient should only be undertaken for emergencies.

There is a theoretical risk that anaesthetic agents may be teratogenic if a pregnant woman is exposed in early pregnancy, but there is little if any statistical evidence to support this. Whilst it makes sense to avoid giving anaesthetics to pregnant women if this can be avoided, there is no evidence of risk to personnel working in operating theatres, at least in today's scavenged theatres. Many anaesthetists continue working to a quite advanced stage of pregnancy.

The Nervous System

Convulsions

Convulsions may occur in the post-operative period for the same reasons as they may occur on the medical ward. Amongst the avoidable causes are the use of potentially convulsant drugs such as methohexitone and enflurane in known epileptics, and the administration of an overdose of local anaesthetic. Stroke occurs and can precipitate convulsions, and there are 'metabolic' causes of convulsions such as hypoglycaemia, hyperpyrexia and eclampsia. It follows that any patient having a convulsion requires, among other things, to have a blood sugar estimation.

The management of post-operative convulsions follows the same principles as that of convulsions in any situation: supportive treatment (including maintenance of the airway), treatment of any causative factor (such as hypoglycaemia) and administration of specific anticonvulsants such as benzodiazepines.

Delayed Recovery

This annoys recovery room staff and worries relatives but in the vast majority of cases is due simply to a relative sensitivity to anaesthetic agents or a relative overdose of drugs such as opioids. Patience is a virtue in these circumstances, although it must be stated that one of the authors has had to wait four days for a patient to recover to a reasonably alert state!

Occasionally, delayed recovery is a manifestation of a more sinister event. Strokes and myocardial infarction may present in this way, and it may be the first sign of an endocrine disorder such as diabetes or thyroid under- or over-activity. Finally, the patient who is hypoxic or shocked will suffer delayed recovery.

Intraoperative Awareness

This is listed here as well as in Chapter 1 because, although it occurs during surgery, it will obviously present post-operatively. The important aspect of management, as with any untoward event, is to take the patient seriously and offer a sympathetic, truthful explanation. A proportion of patients who are not given a realistic explanation develop psychological problems which may last for many years. Any patient who complains of intraoperative awareness *must* be seen by a senior member of the anaesthetic staff, who will listen to the history, investigate the cause, reassure the patient and arrange psychological follow-up if necessary.

Extra-pyramidal Side-effects

These occur rarely following the use of anti-emetics such as phenothiazines, butyrophenones or even metoclopramide. Once the (sometimes difficult) diagnosis is made, treatment is straightforward with procyclidine or benzhexol.

Ocular Complications

Corneal abrasions may occur if the eyes are left open, and are a particular risk if the patient is in the lateral or prone position or if the face is covered in drapes. Prevention is obvious.

Rarely, diplopia may persist for up to two days when muscle relaxants have been used, and requires simple reassurance.

Peripheral Nerve Damage

This is discussed in Chapter 1. Patients particularly at risk are those with a subclinical neuropathy such as diabetics, alcoholics and patients with rheumatoid arthritis.

Prevention involves the education of all those involved in patient transfer and positioning so that they are aware of the risks. Should nerve palsy occur, the patient should be reassured that recovery will take place, although it may take weeks or months.

Problems of Temperature Control

Patients inevitably become slightly hypothermic during surgery. A fall in core temperature of 1°C or so is almost unavoidable during anaesthesia, even if precautions such as use of a blood warmer, warming mattress and humidification of inspired gases are taken. Neonates are a particular problem and require a warm operating theatre and special attention to temperature of skin preparation fluids and so on.

What problems are associated with this form of accidental hypothermia? Obviously if the temperature falls to 32°C or below then there is a significant risk of cardiac arrest. Even lesser degrees of hypothermia pose a risk because rewarming requires increased oxygen consumption (exacerbating hypoxia) and increased cardiac output (stressing the ischaemic or failing heart). It follows that patients with respiratory or cardiac disease require extra attention to temperature conservation during anaesthesia.

At the other extreme, malignant hyperthermia may present in the recovery room or even after return to the ward. The rise in temperature must be distinguished from that associated with sepsis or thyroid crisis. The biochemical changes of malignant hyperthermia are usually diagnostic.

Minor Aches, Pains and Trauma

The following complications are described as 'minor' to contrast them with the potentially harmful complications described above. It is not intended as a dismissive term since these problems may be very distressing to the patient.

Sore Throat

This occurs after up to 50 per cent of general anaesthetics. Tracheal intubation is often a contributing factor but is not the only one because breathing dry gases for more than a very brief period causes sore throat. This problem usually resolves within 24 hours.

Headache

This occurs after 15–35 per cent of general anaesthetics and is more common after minor surgery. The aetiology is unknown but again it normally resolves within a few hours.

Laryngeal Granuloma

This should be considered if hoarseness persists for longer than about a week after an anaesthetic involving tracheal intubation. It is particularly distressing for those, such as opera singers, whose livelihood depends on their voice. For others, such as British Rail announcers, it may be a positive advantage in their career!

Suxamethonium Myalgia

This is the proper term for the muscle pains which occur following the use of the muscle relaxant suxamethonium (see Chapter 3). They occur particularly in young, active patients who resume normal activities soon after surgery and so tend to occur most after day-case surgery. The best way to prevent them is to avoid the use of suxamethonium, but this is not always possible.

Trauma to Teeth

This complication should occur rarely if tracheal intubation and airway maintenance are performed properly. It is more serious if the dislodged tooth or crown passes into the bronchial tree and needs to be retrieved broncho-scopically.

Surgical Complications

The anaesthetist may also become involved in post-operative problems which are, strictly speaking, 'surgical'. Major haemorrhage may require the assistance of those experienced in resuscitation from severe hypovolaemia. In addition, anaesthetists have now assumed the responsibility for treatment of acute pain following surgery (see Chapter 7).

Key Points

- No anaesthetic is totally without complications.

- Many of these complications are unavoidable, but it is still important to reduce their incidence and severity to a minimum.

- Alertness to the potential complications of a technique will aid prevention.

- A high index of suspicion will assist rapid diagnosis of these problems and allow prompt treatment.

- The responsibility of the anaesthetist extends beyond the operating theatre and recovery room into the surgical ward and (in the case of day-stay surgery) into the patient's home. The anaesthetist needs to be aware of the long-term consequences of anaesthetic techniques, both because he or she may be able to help with treatment and for self-audit purposes.

Further Reading

Taylor, T.H., Major, E. (eds) 1993: *Hazards and complications of anaesthesia*. Edinburgh: Churchill Livingstone.

9 Intensive Care

Introduction

The specialty of intensive care is concerned with the support of failing physiological systems (e.g. respiratory, cardiovascular, renal). Historically, it derives from the units set up for ventilation of paralysed patients during the poliomyelitis epidemics of the early 1950s. Those 'respiratory units' consisted of rows of medical students squeezing bags in shifts, a far cry from the modern automatic ventilator with its knobs, dials and flashing lights.

Some intensive care units (ICUs) are run by non-anaesthetists. However, anaesthetists' familiarity with artificial ventilation and cardiovascular physiology, together with their experience of liaison with other specialties, makes them the most usual source of intensive care specialists.

Most hospitals have a 'general' ICU which admits critically ill patients from all parts of the hospital. There may also be a more specialized ICU such as a burns unit, cardiac surgery unit or paediatric ICU. Some coronary care units may be regarded as ICUs.

Patients admitted to ICU require meticulous attention to all their physiological functions. A ratio of one nurse to one patient is common, and an intensive care specialist (consultant or trainee) is immediately available. Intensive monitoring is used, and action taken quickly if physiological variables change significantly.

Categories of Patient Admitted to the Intensive Care Unit

These are summarized in Table 9.1. They are most conveniently divided into single-organ failure, multiple organ failure and 'precautionary' admissions (where problems are foreseen with a specific patient and the ICU is regarded as a safer place for these problems to arise than a general ward).

Whatever the reason for the patient's admission, the severity of the condition may be graded by one of a variety of 'scoring systems'. These seek to define the degree of physiological derangement and thereby predict the likely outcome. The best known is APACHE – an acronym for applied physiology and chronic health evaluation. This fairly self-explanatory phrase describes a system for combining scores for the severity of the acute

Table 9.1 Examples of types of patient admitted to the intensive care unit

1. Single organ failure

   (i) Respiratory failure
   see Table 9.2 for causes
   (ii) Cardiovascular failure
   cardiogenic shock
   after cardiac surgery
   overdose of cardiac depressant drugs such as beta-blockers
   (iii) Renal failure
   following prolonged hypotension or shock
   (iv) Gastrointestinal failure
   for initiation of parenteral feeding following, for example, extensive bowel resection
   (v) Neurological failure
   following major head injury or prolonged neurosurgery

2. Multiple organ failure

   (i) Multiple injuries (head, chest, abdomen, etc.) following road traffic accidents or similar trauma
   (ii) 'Sepsis syndrome' — a term used to describe the combination of cardiac, respiratory, renal and often gastro-intestinal failure occurring as a consequence of septicaemia
   (iii) 'Shock syndrome' — a combination of organ system failures similar to the sepsis syndrome, but occurring following prolonged, profound shock

3. 'Precautionary' admissions

   (i) Following major surgery, e.g. major thoracic surgery or major vascular surgery
   (ii) Following any surgery on high-risk patients, e.g. patients with cystic fibrosis or congenital heart disease
   (iii) Occasionally, for observation of patients with progressive 'medical' conditions such as status asthmaticus or neurological disease (Guillain-Barré, etc.)

physiological derangement with scores for the patient's 'pre-morbid' condition. Thus, for a given acute situation the outcome is likely to be worse if the patient already suffers from, for example, coronary artery disease or diabetes.

It is debatable whether there should be any absolute exclusion criteria for ICU admission. It is normally considered inappropriate to subject patients with terminal malignant disease to the discomfort and indignity which may be associated with intensive care procedures in order to extend life by a few days or weeks. Age is less of a barrier than it used to be, and patients in their eighties are nowadays admitted to ICUs. When patients have other chronic disease, the quality of life becomes an inevitable consideration, and this of course is a matter of subjective interpretation for the patient, the family and ICU staff.

General Intensive Care Management

Nursing Care

The high ratio of nurses to patients has already been mentioned. The nurse must be trained to understand the significance of changes in monitored variables and to observe the patient for other changes – restlessness, anxiety and so on – which cannot be measured by monitors. The nurse must communicate with the patient, however unconscious the patient appears to be, and carry out all the tasks required for a comatose patient.

Infection Control

All patients on an ICU are at risk of hospital-acquired infection. Surveys show that up to 40 per cent of patients acquire an infection during their ICU stay, and this figure is of course higher in patients who are immunocompromised, which many are.

Aseptic precautions must be meticulous. Insertion of cannulae for monitoring and treatment, management of urinary catheters and other invasive devices, and other manoeuvres must all be carried out as aseptically as possible. Doctors and other personnel should wash their hands between treatment of each patient, and attention must be paid to potential reservoirs of infection (this is why vases of flowers are rarely seen on ICUs).

Many ICUs have strict protocols for the use of antibiotics, to prevent the development of resistant strains of bacteria, and close liaison is maintained with the microbiology department.

Sedation and Analgesia

Most patients admitted to an ICU require artificial ventilation or some other uncomfortable procedure. Nearly all require sedation at some stage of their stay. Benzodiazepines are commonly used, but there has recently been a move towards the use of infusions of intravenous anaesthetics such as propofol. Requirements for sedation normally decline during a patient's stay so that, for example, many patients tolerate artificial ventilation with no sedation at all after a few days.

Sedation must not be used as a substitute for analgesia. ICU patients are frequently in pain following surgery or trauma, and these patients tolerate procedures better and have less haemodynamic variability if their pain is controlled. Infusions of opioids are commonly used, although epidural analgesia and nerve blocks have an important place in the management of pain.

Problems of Immobility

Immobile patients are at risk of a number of complications, such as decubitus ulcers ('pressure sores') and deep venous thrombosis. Both are even more likely when patients have a low cardiac output. Patient positioning is important, and prophylaxis against thromboembolism should always be considered.

Communication

The ability to communicate effectively is an important attribute of the ICU specialist. The awake or lightly sedated patient requires information and reassurance. ICU staff such as nurses, physiotherapists and doctors in training need accurate diagnosis, an idea of prognosis and guidelines for treatment. Written protocols have an important place here, covering common conditions and emergency situations. They are particularly valuable for ensuring consistency of management when shorter shifts for doctors in training mean that there are many more doctors looking after the patients, and when many ICUs are looked after by more than one consultant.

Communication with patients' relatives is also important. Tactful discussion of a poor prognosis, guarded optimism if the prognosis improves, sympathetic support, or a carefully worded request for organ donation may all be required at different times. These difficult tasks should not be delegated to the most junior member of staff who has little training in, and even less experience of, these matters. Close liaison with fellow clinicians is required.

The majority of patients admitted to an ICU are already under the care of a consultant, and this consultant may rightly have an interest in the patient's management and progress. There will inevitably be times when the ICU management conflicts with that envisaged by the original consultant. This situation needs diplomatic handling to avoid deterioration into unedifying acrimony and poor professional relationships in the future. On a more constructive note, most ICUs maintain a healthy, friendly relationship with other departments such as radiology, microbiology and other 'investigative' departments. Members of these departments frequently take part in ICU ward rounds.

Monitoring in the Intensive Care Unit

General aspects of monitoring are discussed in Chapter 5. Some applications are especially important in intensive care. Continuous monitoring of arterial oxygen saturation by pulse oximetry is almost invariably used, and the critical haemodynamic state of most of these patients is reflected in the fact that many of them have arterial pressure monitored directly from an arterial cannula, as well as central venous pressure or pulmonary artery pressure monitoring. Such continuous monitoring is essential for detecting the sudden changes in arterial and venous pressures which these patients may experience.

These patients are subject to changes in metabolic acid–base status, for example during periods of low tissue perfusion. Frequent estimates of 'arterial blood gases' are required, as this indicates the adequacy of ventilation (by PCO_2), the state of oxygen transfer in the lungs (by PO_2) and the metabolic acid–base state (by base excess and standard bicarbonate).

Support of Individual Organ Systems

The Respiratory System

Some causes of respiratory failure are given in Table 9.2. Occasionally, as with a drug overdose, simple treatment with a specific antagonist is sufficient, but the vast majority of patients with respiratory failure require artificial ventilation. Traditionally, this has been performed in the same way that it is in the operating theatre, with the artificial ventilator completely taking over the patient's respiratory function. More recently, modes of ventilation have been used in which the patient contributes a greater or lesser degree of spontaneous respiratory effort. These techniques have the advantage that

Table 9.2 Some causes of respiratory failure

1. Failure of central drive
   drug overdose
   head injury

2. Failure of neural pathways
   high cervical spine fracture

3. Failure of neuromuscular transmission
   myasthenia gravis

4. Failure of muscle power
   muscular dystrophy

5. Failure cf mechanical support of the lungs
   multiple rib fractures producing a flail segment
   pneumothorax

6. Failure of lung parenchyma
   interstitial pulmonary oedema in, for example, 'shock lung'

7. Failure of alveoli
   frank pulmonary oedema
   aspiration pneumonitis

8. Failure of the airways
   status asthmaticus

9. Failure of pulmonary blood supply
   pulmcnary embolism

the patient requires less sedation, can be 'weaned' from the ventilator more easily and is less disorientated.

Any invasive procedure has its problems. Artificial ventilation requires a tracheal tube or tracheostomy, either of which bypasses the upper airway and so deprives the inspired air of natural humidification and bacterial filtration. Both these factors make lower respiratory infection more likely. In addition, the function of the cilia in the respiratory tract is impaired, and secretions accumulate in the smaller bronchi. Adequate chest physiotherapy is essential.

Any patient who receives positive-pressure ventilation is at risk of 'barotrauma' (lung trauma resulting from positive pressure within the alveoli of the lung), particularly pneumothorax. This may rapidly develop into a tension pneumothorax, one of the most urgent of medical emergencies. Rapid diagnosis and treatment are essential (often there is no time to obtain a chest X-ray) and all ICU staff should be alert to this complication. Pneumothorax is more likely in patients being treated with positive end-expiratory pressure (PEEP), in which the pressure in the lungs is kept above zero in the expiratory phase of the cycle.

A few patients have lungs which are so affected by disease that it is impossible to maintain adequate oxygenation despite a high inspired oxygen concentration and manipulations of the ventilatory pattern such as PEEP (see above). It is sometimes possible to take over the function of the lungs by artificial devices similar to the oxygenator of a heart–lung bypass machine. These devices delight in such acronyms as ECMO (Extra-Corporeal Membrane Oxygenator), in which blood is diverted through a membrane system for oxygen transfer, or IVOX (Intra-Venous OXygenator), in which the membrane function is carried out by a set of branching tubes inserted into the inferior vena cava. The exact role of these devices in the treatment of respiratory failure has yet to be established.

The Cardiovascular System

Many patients arrive in the ICU with low cardiac output, normally (but not invariably) manifested by a low blood pressure. The approach to restoration of a normal cardiac output depends on a consideration of Starling's law of the heart, a relationship well known to medical students and examiners. The clinical application of the relationship is represented graphically in Figure 9.1, which shows that the stroke volume of the ventricle is related to its end-diastolic volume. Expressed more simply, the more blood there is in the ventricle, the more is expelled with each beat (up to a certain limit). The first objective for the patient with a low cardiac output is to ensure that the filling of the left ventricle is optimal. In the more straightforward case this can be achieved by monitoring central venous pressure (CVP) and infusing fluid until the CVP (which represents right ventricular filling) is normalized. When left ventricular function is severely impaired, it is more reliable to titrate fluid infusion against the pulmonary capillary wedge pressure (PCWP) which reflects left ventricular filling more accurately.

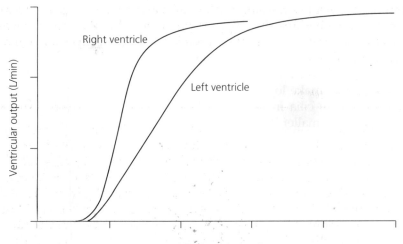

Figure 9.1 Graphical representation of Starling's law of the heart.

This optimization of the circulating volume is often only the first step. Contractility of the myocardium may be impaired by the disease process. Inotropic drugs are those which increase the contractility of the myocardium. They include naturally occurring substances such as adrenaline and dopamine as well as manufactured substances such as dobutamine. The precise properties of each of these drugs determine which will be used in the individual patient, and the details are beyond the scope of this book.

The disease process may affect the peripheral circulation as well as the myocardium, by causing vasodilatation or vasoconstriction. Sometimes vasoconstriction is cured simply by improving cardiac output, as described above. On other occasions it is necessary to administer specific vasodilators (such as sodium nitroprusside or glyceryl trinitrate). If the peripheral circulation is already dialated vasoconstrictors (such as noradrenaline) may be required in order to increase tissue perfusion or alter the afterload of the left ventricle.

This emphasis on the peripheral circulation should not distract us from a consideration of the pulmonary circulation. William Harvey, more than 350 years ago, recognized the importance of the pulmonary circulation, and his description of it as 'the lesser circulation' was not intended to be dismissive. Problems of increased pulmonary vascular resistance occur in cardiac disease (often congenital) and lung disease (congenital or acquired), and may pose considerable problems in intensive care. There are drugs, such as aminophylline, which have a relatively selective effect on the pulmonary circulation, but this is often at the expense of undesirable effects elsewhere. There is current interest in the effectiveness of nitric oxide (NO) (*not* nitrous oxide: N_2O) as a selective pulmonary vasodilator.

Virtually all the drugs mentioned above need to be given by continuous intravenous infusion as they have a short plasma half-life and precise titration of dose is essential. A frequent practical problem for the newcomer to intensive care is simply keeping track of all the infusions which are running into the patient – besides the drugs required for the circulation, there are usually several other drugs such as antibiotics and sedatives as well as the maintenance fluids.

The Renal System

Renal failure in isolation can be dealt with easily on the renal unit by haemodialysis or peritoneal dialysis. However, it is also a frequent component of the multisystem disease which requires intensive care admission, particularly following shock or sepsis. Renal failure then needs to be managed in the intensive care unit. Although the orthodox techniques of haemodialysis or peritoneal dialysis may still be employed, nowadays haemofiltration is used more commonly. This is a continuous process, in contrast to the intermittent nature of dialysis, and causes less disturbance to the circulation than haemodialysis and less variation in lung compliance than peritoneal dialysis.

Haemofiltration, like most intensive care procedures, requires a complicated machine with flashing lights and noises, which of course contributes further to the dismay induced in the senior house officer on his first night on ICU.

The Gastro-Intestinal System

Nutrition is important in intensive care for a number of reasons. At the most basic level, it is impossible for the patient to eat if he has a big plastic tube going through his mouth into his trachea. Many patients have gastro-intestinal failure, either due to ileus following abdominal surgery or due to poor perfusion of the gut in a state of low cardiac output. If anything, adequate nutrition is even more important in intensive care than in the general hospital patient, as wound healing and speed of recovery are known to be related to nutritional state.

In the absence of gastro-intestinal disease, intensive care patients can be fed 'enterally', i.e. by the conventional route. This may be done through a nasogastric tube or, occasionally, through a feeding jejunostomy (in which the food is infused directly into the jejunum). The precise composition of these feeds depends on local custom, but they are always of high nutritional value.

The enteral route should be used if at all possible. If there is gastro-intestinal failure, then the 'parenteral' route must be used and the 'food' infused directly into the vein. This must, of course, contain the usual carbohydrate, protein, fat, minerals, and vitamins but these must already be 'digested' and should ideally be in a solution which is isosmolar and non-irritant. These considerations show why parenteral nutrition is a more complex undertaking than enteral feeding. Add to this the necessity associated with parenteral feeding to carry out frequent blood tests to check electrolyte concentrations (including obscure ones such as copper and zinc), lipid composition and other unusual requirements and it becomes obvious why the enteral route is preferred. One recent improvement has been the development of suitable aseptic techniques in hospital pharmacies to enable the required solutions to be made up locally and supplied in a single large bag – no longer does the intensive care resident have to sit chewing his pencil working out how to provide a patient's individual needs from the variety of solutions available to him.

The Neurological System

Support of the neurological system on intensive care is mainly concerned with the management of severe head injury – which can be taken to mean head injury severe enough to impair consciousness. The physiological problem here is often a state of raised intracranial pressure, and treatment is directed towards reducing this pressure or at least preventing further increase.

Prevention is, as always, the best treatment, and prevention of head injury is particularly important. Legislation on crash-helmets and seat-belts, and safety requirements at sporting events, have all reduced the incidence and severity of head injury in the UK. Anyone doubting the value of such legislation only has to work in parts of the USA. where crash-helmets are not compulsory and the smallest motor-cycle has a 500 mL capacity. The unnecessary damage and death caused to these patients, who are normally young adults, is very distressing to intensive care staff as well as the patient's relatives.

Management of severe head injury aims to prevent the development of further cerebral oedema (which would, of course, increase intracranial pressure further). It is essential to prevent hypoxia, hypercapnia and reduced cerebral perfusion, remembering that these patients are often comatose (increasing the risk of aspiration of stomach contents and hypoxia), have reduced respiratory drive (causing hypercapnia) and may have other major injuries (causing hypovolaemia and reduced cerebral perfusion). It is essential to intubate the trachea at the earliest opportunity (at the scene of the accident if possible), take over artificial ventilation and start an intravenous infusion. Many deaths could be prevented if these simple measures were followed for all patients with severe head injury.

Once on the ICU, artificial ventilation is continued. Other measures to reduce intracranial pressure may be adopted, including administration of osmotic diuretics such as mannitol. The vogue for inducing 'hibernation' with large doses of barbiturate is now over, since it was shown to have no effect on outcome. Steroids are also of no benefit.

It is important to diagnose surgically remediable conditions such as intracranial haematoma or depressed skull fracture. This is done partly on clinical grounds, looking for localizing neurological signs, but mainly by computerized tomography (CT) scan. There is no doubt that the use of regular CT scans has revolutionized the management of these patients – the authors remember the days before CT scans when management depended on a mixture of clinical acumen, experience, guesswork and 'feel'.

There is a specific scoring system for head injuries called the Glasgow Coma Score. This gives a useful index of prognosis, so that relatives can be advised at an early stage, and may also be a useful 'shorthand' for monitoring deterioration or improvement. The use of the intracranial pressure monitor is mentioned in Chapter 5, and may provide a more precise idea of clinical changes.

Many patients with severe head injury are, sadly, potential organ donors. The diagnosis of brainstem death is a clinical one and must follow precise guidelines laid down nationally by the joint medical Royal Colleges. This is probably one of the few instances where no departure from a protocol may be permitted, whatever the circumstances. Whilst many people may regard organ donation as slightly ghoulish, the idea that a premature death has produced some benefit is often reassuring to relatives and ICU staff. The revolution in the life-style of organ recipients is a powerful reminder of the value of these procedures.

The Haemostatic System

Many ICU patients have impaired clotting, either because of massive blood transfusion (bank blood being deficient in clotting factors and platelets) or because the disease process has caused disseminated intravascular coagulation (DIC). Management of these states requires specialist advice from the haematology department, and will involve the use of fresh frozen plasma (FFP), platelets and specific clotting factors. FFP is plasma which is removed from donor blood soon after donation and frozen quickly, thereby preserving the effectiveness of the clotting factors.

Key Points

- The technology of the intensive care unit makes it appear forbidding and incomprehensible to the stranger. Intensive care is, in fact, largely applied physiology and pharmacology and these aspects should be comprehensible to the average second-year medical student.

- Communication is a vital aspect of intensive care. Relatives must be dealt with sensitively, members of staff must be aware of protocols and the plans for each individual patient, and appropriate advice must be sought from other departments such as radiology, microbiology and haematology.

- Intensive care involves the support of failing body systems. Single-organ failure is normally straightforward to manage; the most challenging patients are those with multiple organ failure or multiple injuries.

- The simple aspects of management of these patients are easily forgotten in the heat of the moment and the haste involved in transferring a patient to ICU. Administration of oxygen, setting up an intravenous infusion, and taking standard blood tests, take only a few minutes and can be performed while waiting for a porter to arrive to transfer the patient. Any of these may significantly alter the prognosis of the patient.

Further Reading

Nunn, J.F. *Nunn's applied respiratory physiology.* Oxford: Butterworth-Heinemann.

Tinker, J., Zapol, W.M. 1991: *Care of the critically ill patient.* Germany: Springer Verlag.

Resuscitation

Introduction

It is the recurring nightmare of virtually every newly qualified doctor to be called to attend to an unconscious, apparently lifeless body. This is perhaps less of a worry in hospital practice where help is readily available, but can be dismaying when it occurs in full public gaze, probably at the theatre or a sporting event. It is a reasonable expectation of the public that any doctor should be able to provide at least basic cardiopulmonary resuscitation ('basic CPR'), particularly now that ambulance personnel and increasing numbers of the general public are being trained in the basic skills.

Basic CPR refers to those aspects of resuscitation which can be carried out with no equipment, and has changed little in the last 20 or 30 years. Advanced CPR refers to those aspects of resuscitation which require sophisticated equipment such as an ECG monitor, defibrillator, drugs, tracheal tube and a source of oxygen. This is continuously developing as experience and theoretical knowledge are gained. The European Resuscitation Council and the Resuscitation Council (UK) issue fresh guidelines at intervals, most recently in 1992.

Basic CPR

The mnemonic 'DABC' (Diagnosis, Airway, Breathing, Circulation) should be remembered.

Diagnosis

It is important to establish that the patient has suffered cardiorespiratory arrest and not a simple faint. Shouting at, and gently shaking, the patient will establish that he is unresponsive. Absence of breathing and absence of a major pulse (usually the carotid) confirms the diagnosis and permits the start of CPR. It is advisable to call for assistance at this stage if it is not already available.

The Airway

Sometimes a simple manoeuvre to open the airway, such as elevating the jaw, will allow the patient to restart breathing, and all should then be well.

One of the authors has had to rescue an unconscious skier from the grips of his distraught girlfriend, who was clutching his head to her chest in such a way as to completely obstruct his airway; once her grip was loosened, no further action was necessary!

The treatment of the foreign body in the larynx is a matter of slight controversy. In North America the Heimlich manoeuvre is advocated, in which the rescuer stands behind the patient gripping with both arms round the base of the ribcage and exerts a sudden upwards compression. The foreign body (classically an olive at a cocktail party) is thus forcibly expelled. In the United Kingdom, the approach is for the rescuer to apply blows to the back, clear the airway by sweeping his fingers around the patient's throat and then proceed with resuscitation. The Heimlich manoeuvre may be tried if back-blows fail.

Breathing

Mouth-to-mouth breathing is one of the fundamental skills of medicine. After clearing the airway, elevating the jaw and tilting the head back, the patient's nose is occluded and the rescuer inhales, applies his mouth to the patient's mouth and breathes out, expanding the patient's lungs. Expiration is then allowed to occur passively.

The patient's chest must be watched during this procedure to make sure that it moves outwards when the rescuer breathes into the patient's mouth. If it does not move, then there is probably a problem with the patency of the patient's airway.

This sounds very simple but can be difficult if it has to be performed through a sea of vomit, false teeth and other debris. The Brook airway is now largely of historical interest, but devices permitting mouth-to-mask ventilation help to make things less unpleasant, and so encourage the rescuer. They are shown in Figure 10.1.

Circulation

The first action should be a precordial thump – a sharp blow with the fist or the base of the palm on the base of the sternum. This mechanical stimulus may terminate ventricular fibrillation and allow normal rhythm to resume.

If, as is usual, the precordial thump fails, then the aim is to maintain the circulation by artificial means until normal cardiac activity can be restored by drugs, electricity, or a combination of the two. The cornerstone of this is external cardiac massage. This apparently simple technique was first described as recently as the late 1950s, despite the best efforts of Hollywood film-makers to depict its use by medical heroes at earlier dates.

The apparent simplicity can be deceptive, and it is important to practise the technique properly. The hands are placed one on top of the other over the lowest third of the sternum (see Figure 10.2). The arms are kept straight and pressure is applied through the base of the palms, the aim being to

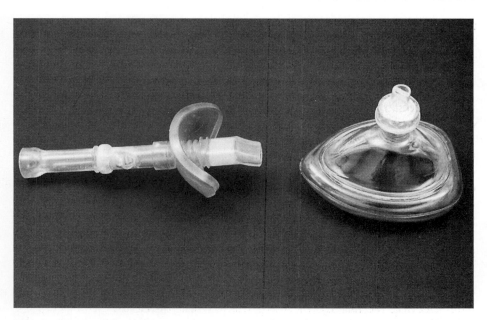

Figure 10.1 Devices used in mouth-to-airway and mouth-to-mask ventilation (Brook airway and Laerdal airway).

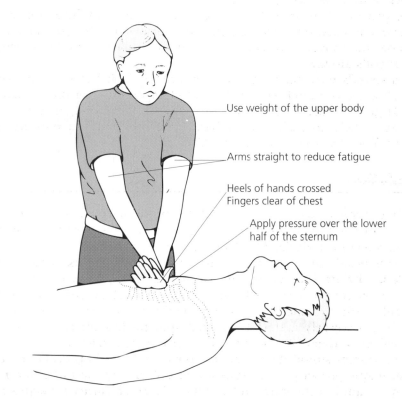

Use weight of the upper body

Arms straight to reduce fatigue

Heels of hands crossed
Fingers clear of chest

Apply pressure over the lower
half of the sternum

Figure 10.2 External cardiac massage.

depress the sternum by 2–3 cm. The frequency of the strokes should be about 80 per minute.

The single-handed rescuer should perform 15 strokes of cardiac massage to 2 expired air breaths. If there are two rescuers, the ratio should be 5 strokes to 1 breath. The reader will have surmised that this activity can be exhausting if prolonged, so two rescuers should work in turns, and each rescuer should take care to perform his tasks calmly and economically. The performer of expired-air breathing should take care against hyperventilation.

Advanced CPR

Once the necessary equipment arrives, resuscitation moves into the advanced phase. Venous cannulation takes place, breathing is taken over by more effective means and normal circulation is restored as quickly as possible.

Breathing

If there is appropriate skill present, the trachea is intubated and ventilation taken over by a self-filling bag ideally attached to a supply of 100 per cent oxygen.

Circulation

The flow-chart shown in Figure 10.3 should be followed as it shows the guidelines of the Resuscitation Council (UK). An ECG diagnosis is essential. The rhythm may be one of three: ventricular fibrillation (irregular, unco-ordinated wave-like activity of the ventricle), asystole (no electrical activity) or electromechanical dissociation (normal electrical rhythm but no cardiac output).

TREATMENT OF VENTRICULAR FIBRILLATION

This relies upon electrical defibrillation, which interrupts the random activity in cardiac muscle, enabling electrical activity to be transmitted from normal pacemaker tissue, with resumption of normal rhythm. Defibrillation should be performed according to the cycle shown in Figure 10.3. Adrenaline is given during each cycle to ensure that the myocardium remains sensitive to the electrical stimulus.

TREATMENT OF ASYSTOLE

Defibrillation is attempted initially in case fibrillation has been missed. Adrenaline is again used to stimulate electrical activity, and a high dose of atropine given to block the vagus nerve completely. The aim is either to restore normal rhythm or to create ventricular fibrillation which can then be defibrillated.

ADVANCED CARDIAC LIFE SUPPORT

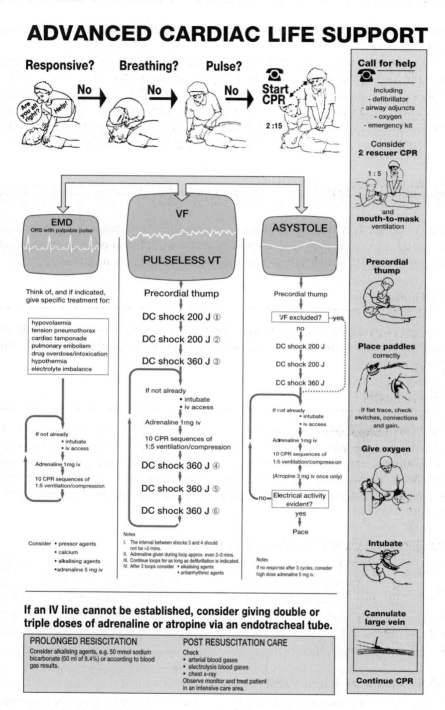

Figure 10.3 Guidelines of the Resuscitation Council. © Copyright ERC 1992, from *Resuscitation* vol 24, 111–21.

TREATMENT OF ELECTROMECHANICAL DISSOCIATION

An underlying cause such as hypovolaemia or tension pneumothorax should be sought and treated. If none can be identified then the outlook is dire. Adrenaline is worth a try.

It is obvious from this account that only two drugs need to be used during early CPR – adrenaline and atropine. Other agents such as anti-arrhythmics and inotropic drugs may be needed following resuscitation, but there is no need to agonize over choice of drugs during resuscitation.

Prolonged Resuscitation

If CPR is prolonged, it may be necessary to treat the inevitable metabolic acidosis by administration of small quantities of sodium bicarbonate. Ideally this is titrated against the results of arterial blood gas measurements but samples for blood gas analysis are difficult to obtain in a pulseless patient. A large central vein should be cannulated if the practitioner is sufficiently skilled. Cardiac massage and ventilation must, of course, be continued throughout.

It is difficult to judge when to abandon attempts at resuscitation. The age and overall condition of the patient must be taken into account, and also the cause of the cardiac arrest. Victims of drowning, hypothermia and drug overdose have been resuscitated successfully after several hours of cardiac massage. Each case must be treated on its merits. Dilated pupils are an unreliable indicator of prognosis.

Post-resuscitation Care

Following successful resuscitation, the patient will require a period of close observation. Often this will be on an intensive care unit but if the patient is breathing normally and is conscious then a coronary care unit may be appropriate.

A number of investigations are essential. A chest X-ray may show, amongst other things, evidence of aspiration of stomach contents (a common occurrence during cardiorespiratory arrest), rib fractures caused by vigorous cardiac massage and the position of the tracheal tube if this is still present. Measurement of plasma electrolyte concentrations may help to identify the cause of the cardiac arrest and reveal the effect on plasma potassium concentration of any adrenaline which has been given. Arterial blood gas analysis identifies metabolic acidosis resulting from the low cardiac output, and hypoxia which may result from lung contusion or aspiration.

A significant proportion of patients who are resuscitated successfully die before leaving hospital. On average, 30–40 per cent of patients can be resuscitated initially but only 10–20 per cent survive to leave hospital. The exact figures depend on the case-mix of the hospital, whether the cardiac arrest is witnessed or not, the cause of the arrest and many other factors. The apparently low success rate is not intended to discourage attempts at resuscitation – far from it, because there are very few medical interventions in which success can be so rewarding.

Selection of Patients for CPR

It is clearly inappropriate and callous to subject all patients to the trauma of CPR before they are allowed to die. Many patients should die peacefully and with dignity. Of course, it is not the function of the cardiac arrest team to decide within a few seconds whether a specific patient should be subjected to CPR. That decision should be taken by a senior member of the patient's medical team, after discussion with the nursing staff and with the patient and family. The decision should be recorded clearly in the medical and nursing notes so that no-one is in any doubt. It may sometimes be necessary to reconsider the decision.

Factors to be taken into account include the patient's age (although no absolute barrier should be laid down), the likely prognosis of the presenting complaint, and the nebulous 'quality of life', which is difficult to judge and impossible to define. It is almost certainly wrong to resuscitate a dying patient only for that patient to die a few weeks or months later from an inevitably terminal disease.

Education in CPR

As stated above, it is reasonable to expect all doctors to possess at least the basic skills of CPR. In some countries, all hospital employees are required to undergo CPR training and assessment before they are allowed to take up employment, and this regulation applies whether the employee is a cleaner or a Professor of Anaesthesia. Many hospitals in the UK appoint a 'resuscitation officer' to ensure a high level of training amongst the staff.

Increasing numbers of ambulance personnel in the UK are being trained not only in basic CPR skills but also in more advanced skills such as tracheal intubation, venous cannulation, recognition of arrhythmias and defibrillation. Many ambulance services now provide at least one such 'paramedic' on each emergency ambulance.

Often CPR must be initiated by a member of the public, and it is in everyone's interests that as many people as possible are trained in the technique. Cities such as Seattle, USA have pioneered the education of members of the public in basic CPR with considerable success. Health education in its various guises is an established part of the school curriculum in the UK and there is every reason to include CPR training within this subject.

The Future of CPR

The management of cardiorespiratory arrest will change as knowledge and experience advance. It is inevitable that the algorithm shown in Figure 10.3 will change within a few years. Outcome studies may help to determine which patients will not benefit from CPR.

New techniques may become available. The laryngeal mask airway (see Chapter 1) is currently being evaluated as a simpler alternative to tracheal intubation. It may have a place, but is unlikely to replace the tracheal tube as it does not protect the trachea against aspiration of stomach contents.

The (admittedly slow) move towards greater CPR awareness in the population as a whole should be encouraged. The greater the number of people skilled in the technique, the greater the chance of rapid response to an out-of-hospital arrest. This is welcomed by the authors as they look towards their old age!

Key Points

- Every doctor should be skilled in basic CPR and should receive training in intubation and defibrillation.

- Advanced CPR is simply a matter of following the published algorithm.

- The decision as to which patients should receive CPR must be clearly recorded.

- There is a need for greater awareness of CPR amongst the general public.

Further Reading

Baskett, P. 1993: *Resuscitation handbook* (2nd edn). London: Mosby-Wolfe.

Index